So, You're Expecting: Unsolicited Advice from an Uncensored Mother

by Ariana Krum

ISBN 9798880051335

I will start by making the assumption that you are a woman (or family) that is expecting their first baby if you are currently reading this book. First things first: congratulations!! Welcome to the best (and hardest) gang of all: parenthood. And if you are taking the role as Mama Bear, you will soon join the initiation process of a much harder, intense gang to get into – Motherhood. Assuming that you are expecting, I also presume that you were recommended to read a specific book; a book that other women that I know have referred to as "the Bible of pregnancy." Well, let me tell you – as a first-time mother-to-be, that book had a *ton* of great information, but boy did it scare the shit out of me! I also felt like after experiencing my pregnancy with my firstborn, that book did not tell me what *really* happens to us when we are growing a human from scratch inside of our bodies. And most importantly, nobody forewarns you *enough* to sit down, buckle up, and prepare to be humbled… in many ways.

My name is Ariana. I am a mother of two feral boys, twenty-two months apart, currently aged 3.5 years and 1.5 years old. *(I know – what was I thinking!?)* I have three college degrees, in which I gave birth to *both* of my boys while I was obtaining my Master's degree. *(Again, I know – what the actual hell was I thinking!?)* I gave birth to my firstborn at a birth center, unmedicated and natural; this birth was absolutely amazing… the pregnancy, however, was what I could only describe as a personal Hell. With my second son… well, he is often referred to as my Toilet Baby, because he was born at our home right over my toilet, delivered by my midwife! Although his birth was more of a struggle, the pregnancy was a bit easier. It was my pregnancy with my first son, and being recommended to read the afore-mentioned "pregnancy Bible" book that tries telling me what I should expect during my pregnancy that led me to wanting to write this very book. It was like I had every bad symptom that pregnancy has to offer a woman! I also got so sick and tired of women – including my own mother – tell me how easy and smooth their pregnancy was! Because there I was, having Hyperemesis Gravidarum, where I was unable to even hold down water let alone food, feet so swollen that it hurt to walk and no longer able to fit into my super cute Vans shoes, constipated to the brim, and the Conductor of The Crazy Train. "Pregnancy glow" my ass! The only type of pregnancy glow that I experienced was the sweaty aftermath of me vomiting up anything and everything in my stomach! I had absolutely no idea what to expect during pregnancy, let alone where to start. I had to navigate so much by myself – and then COVID reared its ugly head two-thirds of the way through my pregnancy with my firstborn. Talk about a doozy as a new mom.

So, let's begin… I'm going to gently hold your hand and guide you through the twists and turns, from beginning all the way to the end. I don't have much of a filter, and I am probably one of those people that are either loved or hated, so take me with a grain of salt and try not to get too offended. I obviously have my own beliefs and morals that I follow, especially in parenting, but for the purposes of this book and for educating the greater womankind, I will remain unbiased and lay out all research and factual information to the best of my abilities – but be warned: I will touch on the subjects of vaccinations and circumcision. Needless to say, if you are easily offended, close the book or turn off the Kindle now, and forget that you ever let it touch your hands. Pregnancy was scary. Birth was scary. Having a newborn is scary. Being a mother is fucking scary… and I'm just here to remind you, that we are literally all in it together. Like I said – welcome to the gang. Buckle up, honey. The ride has just begun.

Contents

Ch. 1 That "Oh shit, I might be pregnant" moment..................... 1

Ch. 2 The first trimester 7
    The inevitable changes...9
    I confirmed my pregnancy...................................12
    Genetic testing...14
    Growing another organ from scratch?......................15
    Classes to learn how to push.................................18
    The beginning of your medical research..................19
    Cracking your spine while carrying a baby...............19

Ch. 3 Second trimester...23
    More changes to your body.................................25
    Preparing for the baby.......................................25
    Hospital vs. other birthing options.......................27
    Advocate the f*ck for yourself.............................28
    The long-awaited gender reveal............................29
    Anatomy scan..31
    The God-forsaken glucose test............................32

Ch. 4 The end is near – The third trimester....................33
    What to bring to push..35
    Car seat installation and education.......................35
    More research...36
    A plug of mucus... Excuse me? 37
    More testing...37
    Sweeping your membranes 38
    Induce me! 38

Ch. 5 Itsssss baby time! 43
    What does labor feel like?...................................45
    Take this damn pain away! 46
    Labor tips and tricks 49

Checking your cervix during labor.........................51
Implementing your birth plan 52

Ch. 6 The baby has arrived – Now what? 55
After the push 57
The first few days 58
Implementing boundaries others.................................59
Useful crap to have near you 61
Stuff to purchase ASAP..61
Baby's first pediatrician appointment 66
Spoil the baby – But spoil Mom more 66

Ch. 7 After baby arrives: Your new life 69
Postpartum mood disorders.................................71
Who am I now? 72
Paternal postpartum depression 74
Romance after baby 75
Ain't no shame like Mom Shame 76
Daycares – Pros, cons, and assistance.......................76
The controversial topic of sleep training 79

Ch. 8 The first two years 83
Milestones, developments, and signs.........................85
Pesky little phases 87
The "Terrible Twos" 88
"Gentle" Parenting – and "Non-Gentle".....................89

Ch. 9 The [uncensored] expectations of motherhood.............93

chapter one

that "oh, shit, I might be pregnant" moment

I have heard stories about women finding out that they are pregnant from every both ends of the spectrum, and everywhere in between. There was even a television show based around women not knowing that they were pregnant until they just spontaneously gave birth one day! However, I am one of those people that is very in-tune with their body, so when something is even slightly off, I question everything. My symptoms began pretty early; I had extreme indigestion and always felt the urge to burp, which was very weird for me because I quite literally never burp (I will sometimes do this weird hiccup, but I have maybe burped three times in my entire life). I also worked with a coworker which I became close friends with, who said that she was craving spicy food; apparently, she only craved spicy food whenever she was pregnant, or someone close to her is pregnant. After joking around with said coworker at work one day about how I was so gassy and maybe she was craving spicy foods because I was the one that was pregnant around her, I decided to stop at the store on my way home and pick up a pregnancy test… or five. I took a test that evening, and had a positive result. The following morning, I took another, following with another that evening – you know, just to be sure! If I'm remembering correctly, I was supposed to start my period in two days. On the opposite end of the spectrum, I have a friend that personally knows someone that never knew that she was pregnant until she went into labor and gave birth to a baby on her bed in the middle of the day. Insane, right!?

Like I mentioned, my symptoms included indigestion (heartburn and burping), which I knew was out of the norm for me. However, women experience a vast array of symptoms from the beginning! Some women typically experience nausea and vomiting fairly early into a pregnancy (the nausea for me started the following week and just be prepared – it is so, so shitty!). Other symptoms that women could feel early in pregnancy could include breast tenderness and/or enlargement, and fatigue. And let me tell you – if you experience pregnancy fatigue, you just somehow know that it's a very different tired than your normal tired! Now, once you have digested that there could be some weird stuff going on with your body that aligns with pregnancy symptoms, it is time to test! First of all, you should make sure that your period is either missed, or you are only a few days from starting your period, while experiencing any type of pregnancy-related symptoms. Next, the type of test that you choose does not really matter – no matter what anybody says. You can obviously spend the money and buy the fancy pregnancy tests that tell you how many weeks you could be, or what-have-you… but, you could also totally go to your local dollar store and pick up a cheap test, too (these tests just usually entail you having to suck up your urine into a tube and drop it into the test, so make sure to get some gloves at the dollar store too!). If you have not missed your period yet, it is probably best to get a test that shows results a few days sooner than average tests – or you could just be patient and wait a few days for a regular one. Regardless of the test that you end up bringing home and peeing on, the instructions are typically the same and fairly simple to comprehend. If a plus (+) sign shows up, or two double pink lines, that means that you are in fact carrying a child within your womb! There are a lot less hassle with digital tests, as they just give a simple YES or NO. Once you receive any type of indication of a positive pregnancy test, you should start thinking about getting an appointment with your doctor for some bloodwork to confirm the pregnancy. The hormone that pregnancy tests are looking for in your urine is called Human Chorionic Gonadotropin (hCG). This is a hormone that is produced by the placenta, and can usually be traced within your blood or urine within ten to eleven days after conception takes place[1]. Essentially, this hormone will trigger your powerhouse of a body to produce more estrogen and progesterone for the pregnancy; this will allow your uterine lining to thicken, and your body to stop having menstruation[1]. During the first trimester, your hCG levels should continue rising, until about week 10-12, where it will begin to slightly decrease throughout the remainder of your pregnancy. During your upcoming visits with your OB or midwife, your levels will be checked continuously.

I do feel the need to touch on this topic, because nobody told me anything about it: implantation bleeding. Sometimes a woman *will* bleed from the implantation process. This can occur within the first ten to fourteen days after conception, and is pretty common. The process takes place when the fertilized egg attaches to the uterus lining. You can tell the difference between implantation bleeding and your period/a miscarriage because the blood tends to be a pinky-brownish color, and should only be a small amount. Again, nobody told me about implantation bleeding, and when I experienced it after finding out that I was indeed pregnant with my son, you can only imagine how scared I was to find blood when I knew there should not have been any at that point. (Should you experience a darker, more crimson-red color blood while pregnant, please consult a doctor immediately.)

chapter two

the first trimester –
aka, your very own personal hell

Do you know how everyone tells pregnant women that they are glowing? Well, I hate to burst the bubble that you may have of what that glow looks like or is from, but… more than likely, it is caused from the sweat you have dripping down your bloated face from vomiting your entire breakfast up. I swear to you that I have Post Traumatic Stress Disorder when it comes to vomiting, after experiencing Hyperemesis Gravidarum. It was so bad, that I felt nauseous without being around any food, and from being so hungry – and believe me, I was hungry. I would try to drink as much water as I could (as you should during pregnancy), but I wouldn't be able to hold any of it down! I literally survived off of chicken nuggets from Wendy's, and I was only able to eat them in very tiny bunny rabbit bites! I remember cooking dinner one night – chicken, zucchini, and squash in pesto, one of my favorite meals – and I was able to get down to my very last bite… before it all came right back up. Thanksgiving was the worst that year – I was in such a tizzy with my head in the toilet, that apparently, I was not letting everything out fast enough, so stuffing came out of my nose during the process!! And let me just say, pieces of stuffing entering into your sinus cavity is pretty damn painful… and the smell that I had stuck in my nose for a few days after that, entirely turned me off from stuffing (which, again, was a favorite of mine) for about two years! I'm only now starting to eat stuffing again and here I am, in 2024. Some women will experience a lot of nausea and food aversions, whereas others won't experience a single one. Again, every woman's body is different. Your body is different than mine, than mine is from my best friend's body. But, like I said, I was one of those women that got blessed of experiencing all of the shitty symptoms that pregnancy likes to bestow upon us. So there I was – puking up literally air, eating absolutely nothing, but still being so constipated that I felt like I was going to explode. Make it make sense, am I right!?

Not only do you start experiencing symptoms, but you will start to notice your body start to change. Starting first with the bloating! You will literally feel like you look so far along in your pregnancy just from the bloating – but let me assure you, it does usually go away! But I hate to break it to you… you might find yourself going shopping for some larger pants. And let me give you the best piece of advice that I think I will offer in this entire book: go ahead and buy the maternity pants *now*. You will thank me later. Those beautifully designed pants give you so much room, but allow you to still feel stylish! And nobody knows the wiser yet!! Plus, they will last you throughout your pregnancy more than likely! And the amount of peeing you will do throughout the duration of your pregnancy… phew, just get ready to use the bathroom more than you ever have in your entire life! Make sure to use the bathroom before you leave to go anywhere, when you get somewhere, and before you leave that place! Your boobs will also (more than likely) start to grow bigger, and will also probably be a bit tender to the touch. I wasn't able to wear any super restricted bras during my pregnancy with my firstborn because of how tender my girls were! And, just for safe measures, I will forewarn you to not get excited about your boobs not being tender or sore anytime soon, because the process of your milk coming in after giving birth is one son-of-a-bitch, even if you decide not to breastfeed! There are other changes occurring outside of the physical changes – and I'm talking about the emotional and mental changes. Like I had said previously, I was the Conductor of The Crazy Train. And if you ask the father of my children, he will without a single ounce of hesitation agree with the statement. The way that your emotions change during pregnancy… it's indescribable. It's almost as like you feel as though you have zero control over your emotions. And it's the suckiest feeling ever. You get so mad, sad, happy, scared… for no reason! I mean, there might be actual legit reasons that you would be upset, but pregnancy only intensifies those emotions. A situation where you would normally be cool, calm, and collected, and waited to weigh out your emotions before responding, pregnancy hormones get you heated and emotional right there in the moment, causing you to look like a crazy bitch that just wants to control everything. When in reality, the only thing you actually want to control is your own damn emotions! This was probably my biggest hurdle outside of the physical ailments of pregnancy to conquer. I am typically a very independent woman; I do not like relying on people for things, and I have never been one much for strong PDA with my partners. But, during pregnancy, you can only guess what happened… the exact opposite. I felt like the neediest woman alive! I needed so much reassurance and love and kindness displayed towards me, or it made me feel like I was unwanted, period. With your changing body, your self-conscious sometimes starts playing tricks with you; try your best not to let the intrusive thoughts win, because in reality, you look better than you feel. Plus, you *are* growing a human from scratch – and that is a freaking superpower, so you should totally feel like a bad bitch anyway!

Next up: scheduling your first ultrasound appointment. And I suppose that I could kind of tie this in with finding your OBGYN, or researching alternative methods of giving birth. The obvious choice would be going through your insurance and finding a provider that accepts your insurance plan; however, there are other providers available when it comes to delivering a baby, and they may even accept your insurance! I have always had the vision that I wanted to have a natural birth when I got pregnant, even before I met the father of my children. I had listened to stories that my mother told me about a very long needle going into her back when she was laboring, and in the middle of a contraction having to stay still while the needle went into her spine nonetheless! NO thank you!! I would much rather go through the pain of labor than having to go through something like that (and I say this having sat through an eight-hour tattoo in one session). Then I began doing the research about epidurals, and that began my quest into learning more about the birthing world in general. I had a few friends at that point in my life that had children, and one specifically that I will forever hold responsible for cementing in my decision about home births, after sharing her birth story of her daughter with me. The way that she described it all – it was like this beautiful connection with her body, self, and baby; it was described as nothing but divine love. Anyway – you should ask yourself how you see yourself giving birth, and where. Do you prefer a hospital, where there are medical devices to assist in case of an emergency? Do you prefer a staff of doctors and nurses nearby? Do you find peace and solace in your home and see yourself giving birth in your bedroom? It is all about what *you* want, and are comfortable with. Although I knew that I wanted a natural birth at home, it was my and my partner's first child, so we toured the hospital that I would most likely deliver my baby at. I was very early in my pregnancy, and I just remember the anxiety that I felt during the tour; although I was not exactly for having my son in a hospital, I agreed to begin seeing the OBGYN that delivers at the hospital. All was going well, but as I mentioned before, COVID hit when I was six months pregnant.

I Confirmed My Pregnancy… What Do I Do Now?

Knowing the next steps once you find out you are pregnant are a bit of a nuisance, I'm not going to lie. First things first: finding an OB and/or midwife, as I mentioned previously. Go through the steps of finding a provider that accepts your insurance (or not!), and let them know that you just found out that you are expecting, and need to schedule your first prenatal appointment. Not all providers do the exact same thing at the initial appointment, but you should probably expect a full medical history review, checking vitals, giving a urine sample, confirming pregnancy again, a physical which includes a breast exam, and possibly even an ultrasound to check on the growing baby! Your provider should discuss your medical history, including your last menstrual cycle, gynecological history, and any past pregnancies. You should be completely honest in the details that you provide, including any medication that you may be taking (including vitamins and supplements). I would also be sure to be honest about your lifestyle – such as using tobacco products (cigarettes/vapes), alcohol, caffeine, and any recreational drugs (yes, even if you have your medical marijuana card). Speaking of your medical marijuana card – I would make sure to speak to your OB/midwife about your usage and be advised accordingly by professionals while pregnant. At the initial prenatal appointment, your due date will also typically be discussed. I want to tell you what I had to learn myself: your due date is nothing but a guestimate of when the baby may choose to come. The due date is based off of your menstrual cycle, but my own experience had me with literally four different due dates for my firstborn at one point (and ultimately, he came out at 37 weeks anyway!). You should *not* rely heavily on your due date – unless, of course, you choose to schedule a C-section for any given reason and have an actual day scheduled to give birth! And that is a whole entire other topic that you should be discussing with your provider: scheduled C-section and/or inductions. The most important takeaway that I want my pregnant readers to get from this book, from my words, as a new parent is to *research everything*. Ask questions about everything, even if you think you already know the answer. Ask five people the same question. Gather data, do your research, before making a decision about anything regarding you and your baby. Learn about inductions: the process, the risks, others' experiences. Although doctors were ultimately meant to guide patients in the right direction pertaining their health, it is our responsibility to ourself and our babies to do the work ourselves, and know what it is that we are being told and/or recommended. Now do not skew my words – I am in no way telling you to go against doctors' orders… All I am *suggesting* is doing your own research before making any permanent decisions. Another thing that will probably happen at your first prenatal appointment is some bloodwork; this, again, confirms your pregnancy, but checks your hCG levels, detects any other potential infections, measures your hemoglobin, and verifies your blood type. Once this visit is all done and over with, you should expect your next visit to be scheduled for about another month out, and up until pretty much the third trimester, they will continually be spaced out about a month apart. (Once you get into your third trimester, they usually go to every two weeks, depending on your provider's recommendations.)

Genetic Testing – Not Diagnostic Testing

At one of your earlier prenatal appointments, usually between six to ten weeks along, you will be screened for any congenital conditions (such as trisomy 13, Down syndrome, and spina bifida). Now, let me get one thing straight right now – this testing is *entirely optional*. What they do not tell you, is that this only tests the baby's genetics, and is not a diagnosis. To see if the baby does actually have any genetic abnormalities, you would need to undergo a different, more intrusive kind of test, where they have to actually test the baby while in the womb. The genetic test that is done during your prenatal appointment is only to tell you whether you, Mom, are a *carrier* for the gene. And, if you remember anything at all about biology from school, you would know that each human being is composed of 46 chromosomes (the things that contain DNA), which are actually 23 *pairs* of chromosomes! So, I will use my genetic test results that I had done with my firstborn as a comparison here. I tested positive as a *carrier* for spina bifida. What does that mean for my baby? It means that without knowing whether or not Dad is a carrier, the baby has a 25% of being a carrier of spina bifida. Now, let's say that Dad tested positive to being a carrier for spina bifida as well; that would then mean that the baby would have a 50% chance of being a carrier. When my OB office called to tell me the results (yes, they *called* me with this news), it sent me into an anxiety-ridden spiral at work, to the point that I had to ask to go home for the remainder of the day. There is not a lot of explanation behind the genetic testing, and I feel like women get scared senseless because it is not explained properly to them, or they do not go home and do their own research to (try to) answer any questions. So, should you choose to have the genetic testing done, I would recommend two things: 1, take a deep breath and try to remember that this is not a diagnostic test for the baby, and 2, should you get a positive result for a genetic disorder, and you are concerned about the baby being a carrier, get Dad tested as well. Furthermore, if Dad tests positive for being a carrier, seek your provider's professional advice regarding advanced testing. Anyway… Back to the topic at hand here. Normal genetic testing includes an AFP screening, estriol, inhibin, and again, hCG[2]. An AFP screening tests the amount of alpha-fetoprotein (AFP) in your blood during pregnancy; this is a protein produced by the fetal liver and is present in the amniotic fluid[2] (the fluid that surrounds your baby in the womb). This test is used to identify any chromosomal abnormalities or open neural tube defects; this test can also actually determine twins! As I mentioned, there are other more in-depth testing that can be done should there be any abnormalities identified and/or the parents want to have further testing conducted. Although the information is available, I would rather that women seeking further testing related to genetic abnormalities consult their provider for further available options, as it usually varies what is available/offered.

While you are growing a human from scratch in your
womb, you will also be growing another organ. This organ is *the*
life-line for your baby. This magical, beautiful organ is called the
placenta. The placenta will provide your baby with nutrients and
oxygen throughout the duration of the pregnancy. The placenta
also helps rid of waste products from the baby's blood. And when
it is time to give birth to your baby, you will first birth the baby,
and then birth the placenta (also referred to as the "afterbirth").

The placenta will form in one of two positions inside your
womb alongside the baby. You will either have an anterior
placenta, or a posterior placenta. A posterior placenta is when the
placenta has attached to the back of the uterus, whereas an
anterior placenta is when the placenta attached to the front of the
uterus. In normal terms, with an anterior placenta, it will be:
belly, placenta, baby; with a posterior placenta, it will be: belly,
baby, placenta. Women that have an anterior placenta will
typically not feel the baby start kicking until about twenty-ish
weeks, however women with a posterior placenta are able to feel
the baby kicking and moving around twelve-ish weeks along.
Knowing the position of the placenta versus baby will help you in
the long run, because it will help you (kind of) determine how
labor pain will go for you. Personally speaking, I have had both
positions of placenta during my two pregnancies; my oldest had a
posterior placenta, while I had an anterior placenta with my
youngest. From experience, the labor that I had with my
youngest (anterior placenta – belly, placenta, baby) was much
more painful, because it was all within my lower back area. With
my oldest, a lot of my labor pain was felt in my lower belly and
uterus area. Regardless of placement, the placenta will be birthed
shortly after the baby makes its grand arrival.

I feel the urge to also forewarn pregnant women that the
placenta is just as valuable and fragile as your baby. This organ is

literally your baby's lifeline while in the womb. There *are* things that can go wrong in your pregnancy caused by your placenta. For example, I had a friend that was pregnant the same time as I was with my second (this was her fourth, so definitely seasoned!), and we ended up having the same due date. Well, one day as she was loading her big ass stroller into her van when she was about twenty-eight weeks pregnant, and she said she felt something feel as though it ripped inside of her and if I'm not mistaken, had began bleeding shortly thereafter. When she went to the hospital, she found out that she had a placental abruption… when the placenta begins to come away from the wall of the womb (and needless to say, the baby came much earlier than expected and had quite the battle ahead of him). There are other instances when the placenta can unfortunately be a foe instead of a friend during your pregnancy; there are five potential insufficiencies to be aware of: preeclampsia, placenta previa, placenta abruption, and placenta accreta spectrum[3]. Many times, an ultrasound or a "stress test" can detect any fetal insufficiencies. Preeclampsia is the pregnancy complication which results in the mother having high blood pressure and potential kidney damage; signs of this would include very rapid weight gain, swelling in your fingers and/or legs, and headaches. Keep a close eye on your blood pressure and your weight gain, specifically. Whenever the cervix is partially/fully blocked by the placenta is when placenta previa occurs. Unfortunately, this can be a problem when it comes time to deliver the baby, as it can block the baby from lowering into the cervix to be birthed. Symptoms typically include cramping and bleeding, usually after the 20-week mark of pregnancy[3]. Women can usually resolve the issue themselves, by restricting themselves in activities (yes, including sex), resting their pelvis, and possibly medication. On the other end of resolving the issue, if the placenta does not move, you may have to undergo a C-Section. Me being me – I looked into why women sometimes experience placenta previa; and unfortunately, there is no for-certain cause – but, research has found that it could has been often related to women that has previously given birth, has uterus scarring, or carrying more than one baby[3]. (Also, it has been found mostly in non-white women over the age 35, and in patients that regularly smoke or use cocaine[3].) And, as my friend had, placenta abruption occurs whenever the placenta has begun to prematurely separate itself from the uterine wall[3]. Should this happen, it is *very* dangerous to both the baby and Mom; it could cut off the baby's oxygen supply, restrict nutrients from the baby, or prompt a premature/stillbirth delivery[3]. Placenta abruption is not something that just happens – it typically occurs whenever Mom experiences some type of physical trauma, like falling or a hard hit to the abdomen. Also, another causation could be attributed to a rapid loss of amniotic fluid[3]. On the flip side of placenta abruption, there is placenta accreta spectrum; this happens when the placenta gets way too comfy on the uterine wall and wants to expand into the uterus (the placenta could go as far as reaching the bladder, or wrapping around the rectum!). There is no real way of detecting whether or not this is occurring during pregnancy, as the issue with this is that the placenta refuses to budge after the baby is born. Sometimes the placenta, or parts of it, wants to hang on and live on in the womb without the baby… and removing it could cause a substantial amount of blood loss for Mom. Unfortunately, if this were to happen, it could lead to a hysterectomy being done. Other conditions related to the placenta that women should be aware of is placenta increta, where the placenta invades the uterus' muscles, and placenta percreta, which occurs when the placenta actually grows *through* the uterine wall[3].

Classes to Learn How to Push a Baby Out of You

Typically, and especially for first-time mothers/parents, providers offer birth classes. Should you choose to go down the route of a birth center/home birth and have a midwife on your birth team, they usually offer their patients birth classes. However, a quick search on the Internet could find you some local pregnancy support groups, which sometimes include birth classes. You can also ask your local hospital, or even family and friends. It would also benefit to look into local pregnancy centers within your vicinity; there is also the option of private childbirth education organizations. Whichever way you may find a birth class – even if it is on your own time utilizing YouTube videos – I would definitely cut out some time of your schedule to attend most, if not, all of them. I had attended the birth class offered by my midwife and her center, and learned so much that helped me get through the pain of a natural labor and delivery; but I was a dumbass the second time around and chose not to attend any birth classes, and needless to say, I had a much different experience with that labor and delivery. Now, I am not saying that birth classes will teach you how to just ignore the pain of labor, or how to push a baby out (because in the moment of giving birth, all of that information kind of leaves your brain anyway), but I will say that it the classes offer you more knowledge about how to make yourself more *comfortable* during labor, and making it much more tolerable. Classes also offer your spouse/partner support, and teaches them how to best support you and make you as comfortable during labor as well. Most birth classes will also offer assistance with siblings, and even postpartum care. (Also, if you are choosing a natural birth, I highly recommend looking into "hypnobirthing.")

The Beginning of Your Medical Research

The beginning of your medical research as a parent should start *now*. With yourself. Learning about the different medical testing and/or vaccinations that pregnant women are recommended to undergo should be a priority to becoming an educated mother and parent. During your pregnancy, you will be recommended to get vaccines, including the Tdap vaccine and the flu shot. The Tdap vaccine is supposed to help women against whooping cough during pregnancy. In reality, the vaccine reportedly protects women against pertussis (whooping cough), diphtheria, and tetanus. Again, do your research about the vaccine itself, what it prevents, and any other information that you may want to know. Vaccines will be brought up again later down the road, but next time, it will be in regard to your baby. I would highly suggest starting by reading the insert that is required with each vaccine.

Cracking Your Spine While Carrying a Baby (Chiropractic Care)

If you are anything like me, I have been cracking my back since I was a child. I was a gymnast, so every time I would stretch, my back would crack; it just became a consistent habit that lasted the rest of my life (so far). So, when I got pregnant, and the babies started pushing against every single organ of mine, as well as my spine, I was *incredibly* uncomfortable, to say the least. Now, keep in mind that I did not find my midwife until the beginning of my third trimester – so when I started picking her brain about chiropractic care during pregnancy, I was already very large and in charge – and uncomfortable! I did my research, and found that chiropractic care is usually safe for most pregnant woman (if there are underlying health concerns and/or concerns with the pregnancy, chiropractic care should be discussed with a professional and considered very carefully).

I have found that a lot of holistic-y providers will actually recommend getting adjusted during pregnancy, as it helps keep Mom *and* the baby comfy! If the baby is in the breech position (feet down), getting adjusted by a professional could also spin the baby the right way! Also, when I was coming near the end of my pregnancy (mind you, having been told a handful of different due dates so I wasn't entirely sure of when to expect my baby to come), I went to my new prenatal chiropractor for an adjustment, and she was the one that told me that my son would be coming within two weeks… Let me tell you, I had to cancel my standing appointment the following week because I went into labor the day of my appointment! So, getting adjusted actually also helps the baby get more space by moving the head down, *and* get into position, ready for birth! If you start to experience sciatica pain (like I did), getting adjusted will also help relieve some of that pressure and discomfort. But, as with anything you may want to try, I do recommend speaking with your provider before making any decision.

Finding the right provider should be the priority when it comes to beginning your journey into prenatal chiropractic care (if you do not already have a loved chiro that you use, of course). Although most chiropractors are professionally trained to adjust pregnant women, there are chiropractors that have taken specific interests into pre/postnatal chiropractic care; and just like mostly every profession out in the great big world, there is additional training that these chiropractors can take to indulge in their specialty. With pregnancy, your body will be in a constant mode of change, which especially includes your bones and organs! Sometimes women may even experience a misaligned pelvis, which makes delivery a tad bit more difficult. Being adjusted actually has quite a few advantages while being pregnant, like maintaining a healthier pregnancy, controlling symptoms of nausea, reliving back/neck/joint pain, preventing a possible C-Section delivery, and reducing the time of labor and delivery[4]. Did you know, that getting adjusted could actually help you turn a Breech baby!? That's right – there's something that chiropractors use called the Webster Technique; the chiropractor will start by comparing both feet while you are laying on a special pillow on your belly. The chiropractor will bend your legs up towards your booty and assess whether they meet evenly; if not, that could mean that your pelvis is misaligned. Like I said – be careful and do your research before choosing a provider. Remember how I literally just mentioned that there is additional training offered to practitioners? Well, there is a certification program that was launched in 2000 for chiropractors that want to specialize in pre/postnatal (and/or pediatric) care to obtain. The International Chiropractic Pediatric Association (ICPA) is comprised of more than 6,000 chiropractors that have gotten certified[5]. Becoming certified includes the chiropractor attaining 180 hours of additional education that is specific to Webster's methods, and has passed an exam[5]. An internet search could get you a few names of chiropractors that are certified in the specific area, but I would definitely keep it to word of mouth… ask your OB/midwife, or friends, or social media.

chapter three

sailing on smoother seas in the second trimester

More Changes to Your Body

As I had said before, your body will change throughout the entire pregnancy. You should expect a lot of weird shit to happen. Period. I had girlfriends that grew thicker body hair when they were pregnant! During the second trimester, you will begin to notice even more changes to your body. Common symptoms include leg cramps, dizziness, changes to your skin, stretch marks developing, heartburn, swelling, Braxton Hicks contractions, vaginal discharge… the list goes on and on. One of the weirdest things that I began to notice was how I started to have nasal problems. Like, I kid you not, I was either hardly able to breathe, or hardly able to keep the snot from running down my face – and there was absolutely no in-between. There have also been women that have reported dental issues during pregnancy, including losing some enamel. But, along with the bad, is the good! Like *definitely* feeling your baby moving and kicking around! They are no longer flutters that you feel, but full-blown kicks and hooks and jabs and wriggles! It is one of the most amazing feelings that you will experience as a pregnant woman, in my opinion! For me, feeling the baby moving around like a crazy little jumping bean helped me really connect with the growing baby inside of me. It was no longer a fetus or "the baby," but rather, *my* baby… if that even makes sense!

Preparing for the Baby: Choosing What Gifts You Want People to Give You

During the second trimester is a common time for a pregnant woman to begin getting her baby shower gift registry together (if a shower is being held). As a first-time mother, you will literally open Amazon and stop dead in your tracks, not knowing the first thing outside of baby bottles and diapers that you will need. *What kind of crib? What's the safest crib? What is safe sleeping? Will I co-sleep; do I need supplies for that? What size diapers do*

I even get? What size clothes? What if the baby comes early and I need preemie stuff? It's all just a jumble of *what the fuck*. So, first things first: essentials. When I say essentials, I am talking about baby *and* Mom. The baby shower isn't only for the baby; you should be thinking about postpartum care and what you will need *for* the baby (or because of the baby!!) after you give birth. For example, it is obvious that you will need the basics for the baby – crib/bassinet, onesies, diapers, wipes – but what about for Mom? Mom is going to need nipple balm, nursing bras, Epsom salts, snacks, supplements… Things that most people overlook. But not us. Not you. You are going to make sure to add those items onto your baby shower registry! And if anyone asks, you will advocate for your soon-to-be post-giving-birth-to-a-watermelon self and tell them that the baby is not the only one with needs after birth. Now, when it does to come to picking things out for the baby, you have to remember – the baby will more than likely be in your bedroom for the first few months of their life, so you should only buy for the first few months at once. For instance, maybe two boxes of newborn size diapers would last until the baby gained weight (which they do very quickly) and moved up into a size one. You do not need to go overboard with newborn outfits, because the baby, unless is on the smaller side, will only be in that size for a short while. I have watched women go crazy buying ten different types of bottles, not knowing whether the baby will take any of them, or if they will have difficulty with breastfeeding… and it was a waste of money, because they either ended up exclusively breastfeeding, or the baby took to the bottle just fine. Start with one, maybe two, types of bottles and go from there… after the baby is here, though. You will have so many people in your ear, telling you what you do or do not need on your registry – but the bottom line is, you only really need the basics to start out with. Your baby is not going to be using a jumpy seat before they are at least five months old – so you don't need one before the baby even arrives! Take a look at what you really need – and how many of those items you will need; for example, if you plan on bringing the baby to the grandparent's house, put an extra pack and play on the registry!

Hospital vs. Other Birthing Options

As you may have picked up by now, I did not give birth to either of my sons at a hospital. The first baby was born in a birth center, and my second baby was born over the toilet in our home. Although first time parents usually want to give birth at a hospital for the first baby, you should just be aware that there are other options… just as safe as the hospital! The birth center where I gave birth – it was essentially a bedroom setting (with a birth pool, birth chair, etc.) with medical equipment nearby in case it was needed. My midwife and her team had pain relief options on-hand, as well as an emergency plan should anything take a turn for the worst. It helped that the location of the birth center was literally right around the corner from the local hospital, so that was also a nice reassurance. However, what most women/people are unfamiliar with, is a midwife. A lot of people do not know, or perhaps understand, the training that midwives endure to be able to catch babies. To put it in laymen terms, a potential midwife must either complete a graduate program in midwifery, and/or earn their licensure from the American Midwifery Certification Board, or the North American Registry of Midwives[6]. Midwives are more sought after for lower-risk pregnancies; high-risk pregnancies should be cared for by OBGYNs, as they have the surgical training and equipment. Should you choose that you still want a midwife, but to deliver at a hospital, it is more than likely that your chosen midwife will be able to deliver at the chosen hospital, but double check everything just to be certain – and to avoid any mishaps on D-Day!

When it came to my personal decision of where/how I wanted to have my baby, I put a lot of thought into it. For one, I am not the biggest fan of hospitals and get the heebie-jeebies thinking about all of the sickness and germs floating around at any given time, regardless of the amount of sanitizer that is pushed through the ventilation system. Not only that, but I wanted to have control over *my* birth. As it gets shown on the television and in movies, women are usually on the hospital bed, on their back, while giving birth. Considering how our bodies are designed, and where everything is placed – along with the contribution of gravity – lying on your back trying to get something to come down and out of your body is kind of counterproductive. So, I wanted to have the option to be doing a cartwheel giving birth should I so please! And as I mentioned, COVID was big and hitting when I had my first son, so I also did not want to have to be required to wear a mask or get a vaccine or have tests taken, just so that I could safely give birth to my son. So, again, think about *your* desires, comfort levels, and how you ultimately want to bring the baby into this world. *(And not for nothing – but I would also do some research into the cost of birthing a baby at a hospital… because you would be surprised what you would find!)*

*Advocate the F*ck for Yourself… and Your Baby!*

Once you have gotten established with a provider, whether it be a midwife or an OBGYN, you will most likely create a birth plan. Now, let me preface this with – even though you plan it, birth NEVER goes how you expect it. And I think that will remain true throughout parenthood, if I'm being completely transparent. The birth plan will typically have details about how you want to give birth; whether you want pain intervention, and what kind you are willing to get, or if you want skin-to-skin after your baby is born. Your birth plan should include information pertaining to your blood type and emergency contact information. Information related to your labor, birth and delivery, postpartum, and newborn care should all be covered in your birth plan. Again, this plan should only be utilized as an outline, since nobody can predict what will happen while giving birth. You can have your hopes set on having a water birth with your baby, but you may end up having your baby over a toilet! Nonetheless, the birth plan is where you, Mom, will begin advocating for yourself… and your baby. Learn what the process usually entails after giving birth after the hospital, if that is where you will be choosing to deliver; ask them if the baby will ever leave your body, what vaccines are administered, or any other information that you may want to know. Be sure to be bold and loud about things you do not want for yourself or for your baby (I will talk about cervix checks during labor, for example, later in this book).

If you are unsure about your own strength during pregnancy and birth, and/or your amount of support during that time, another idea to plant is having a doula. Basically, a doula is Mom's support; a doula will be the gentle reminder to breathe, repeating affirmations, making sure that you have the support you need whether it is a drink of water or for your back to be massaged. A doula will also help steer your support person into the best direction that helps you. The only downfall with doulas, is that they are not typically covered by insurance – so make sure you do some digging before deciding on one!

The Long-Awaited Gender Reveal

In this section, I feel the urge to touch on a few different topics pertaining to gender. First and foremost, the gender test should have already been conducted by the time you are in your second trimester. But, just know that not every piece of technology or every doctor is right 100% of the time. There are stories out there from women that were told one gender at the ultrasound appointment or their gender reveal party, only for the gender to be quite the opposite when the baby made its grand arrival. So, to cover all of your bases, I would be sure to have a pair or two of opposite-gender or gender-neutral clothing, along with a name for the opposite sex, *just in case*. Secondly, gender disappointment. It is real, and it does indeed suck. If you are totally gung-ho all-or-nothing for a specific gender and you find out that your baby is the opposite gender, you do feel a ping of disappointment. Do not get me wrong – it is not disappointment that your baby is a boy when you were really wanting a girl; it is that you got your hopes up high about it being a girl, and the baby turned out to be a boy. When I was pregnant with my second child, after my son and the hellish pregnancy that I endured with him, I seriously thought that this baby was going to be a girl; the symptoms were different, I felt different, and I even felt like I was carrying different. So you can imagine when it came time to reveal Baby #2's gender, I was fairly surprised that it was in fact a boy and not a girl. As a first-time mother, yes, you are absolutely happy that you have a healthy baby growing inside of you, but finding out the gender is something indescribable. But it *is* something that you get over – and you love your baby not one ounce less regardless of whether the baby turned out to be the gender you had hoped for or not.

That brings me to my next point. Should you find out that you are expecting a bouncing baby boy, the subject of circumcision will more than likely be brought up. This is a fairly controversial subject, as there is a large divide of "wrong vs. right" when it comes to the procedure. Some people believe that the procedure is purely cosmetic and unnecessary, whereas circumcision is actually part of some's religion. So, like I said – pretty large divide. But again, here is something that you should be doing your research on. Find out all of the information you can about how you personally feel about the procedure first and foremost, about your religion and belief system, and about circumcised vs. uncircumcised penises. I know that the father of my children will probably hate that I added this in here, but I am quite literally an open book. My oldest son was circumcised; I went through the entire process with him from start to finish. I had no idea what to expect because I refused to watch any videos of the procedure, but I obviously knew what was being done that day. What I went through as a mother watching what my brand-new baby boy had to go through, and what my son went through during the procedure… I will say, I am glad that our second son is not circumcised. I wish that I could go back in time and change my mind about having my oldest get the procedure done. Because before I started doing my own research into the procedure, I didn't know any better. Now I live by the motto: "Know better, do better." For my second son though, it was a bit different; without getting into too much detail about my son's penis, he was not physically able to have the procedure done. I was also a woman that left that specific decision up to my child's father. However, again, after learning…. Know better, do better. Even if my son was able to have the procedure, I would have completely protested against having it done after knowing what I do now. And just for those that are curious – the procedure actually is solely cosmetic, and there are no health benefits to having it done; also, there is no special way of cleaning an uncircumcised penis either. For further education for yourself, yourwholebaby.org is a very unbiased, informative website for gathering more information on this subject.

Anatomy Scan

The anatomy scan, hands down, has to be one of the most exciting ultrasounds that a pregnant woman looks forward to. Also, one of the most nerve-wrecking ultrasounds. The anatomy scan will go over your baby's anatomy from head to toe. The ultrasound technician will take tons of pictures of your baby, including measurements of its bones and organs. It is so awesome to see, and you will be able to get a much more accurate on how far along you are, and/or a better guestimate of when baby could arrive. This scan will also help your provider determine if there are any defects or issues to be concerned about and/or addressed. The anatomy scan will make sure that your baby's lungs and heart are working properly, and the placenta is doing its job sufficiently as well. Again, knowing the placement of your placenta will help you when it comes time for delivering this watermelon. But, another forewarning for you: your baby's skull *will* look extremely creepy during the anatomy scan but do not fret – your baby comes out much, much cuter!

The God-Forsaken Glucose Test

I will reiterate over and over that there are not enough women that possess the knowledge that they should know when it comes to pregnancy, birth, and postpartum care. Towards the end of your second trimester, you will be approached regarding drinking a special drink to have your glucose levels tested. Now, something that no pregnant woman is actually aware of about this drink, is that it is literally designed to throw your blood sugar levels out of whack. You are consuming an entire bottle of pure sugar essentially. Did you know that you can get exactly what needs to be measured by doing the glucose drink, by drinking a big glass of straight orange juice or apple juice instead? You probably didn't know that – and that's okay, because the doctors aren't going to tell you that. It is up to *you* to request an alternative method. Keep in mind that when they are testing your glucose, they are testing you for gestational diabetes (diabetes that you get while pregnant). If you are downing an entire bottle of liquid sugar that is designed to blow your veins out pretty much, what do you expect the results to read? Again, do your research, and start advocating for yourself!

chapter four

the end is near – the last but not least: third trimester

You probably guessed it – at this point of the pregnancy, you may as well have a Welcome mat down for all of the changes that take place over the nine months. But thankfully, this is the last leg of the pregnancy and the end is *soooo* close now! Your body will begin preparing to deliver the baby. Your back will probably start to hurt even more, your discharge may change a little bit, your baby will lower and get into position, and even the baby's movements may feel different. As your baby begins to descend into the uterus, you will feel a lot more pressure down in your nether regions. While you are in your third trimester, you will probably also begin to feel a lot of pressure in your stomach, which is more than likely gas, and/or even false labor. Also, although you have already been experiencing it, you should probably also expect a touch of even more insomnia!

What Shit Do I Bring to Push a Baby Out?

Let's get one thing straight: you will pack what you need for you *and* the baby. Some things should be very obvious of what to bring and have prepared for when you give birth, like the car seat! For the baby, you will take a few items, but be ready with some room for the stuff that you will take home from the hospital, too! Common items that you would need for the baby includes things like two newborn long-sleeve onesies/pajamas, two short-sleeve onesies, a handful of newborn diapers, formula if you choose not to breastfeed and/or are unable to breastfeed, non-scented baby wipes, and a few bottles. You may want to also include an outfit for the baby if you have pictures at the hospital taken (or a "going home" outfit). Now, for Mom, the items look a little bit different. Things packed for Mom should include things like comfy clothes (sweats/pajamas), a warm robe, makeup of your desire, extra hair ties, glasses/contacts, phone charger, and snacks! I would also advise on slipping some of those packets that are made for your water that adds extra electrolytes; I know that after my second son, I absolutely lived off of a nice cold water with some added Liquid IV. For snacks, I would make sure to add in some higher protein snacks.

Car Seat Installation and Education

Something that I have become very passionate about learning and educating other mothers about, is car seat safety. The very first point of instruction that should be taken in regard to safely installing the car seat, should be taken directly from the car seat's safety manual. The manual will provide you with every ounce of information that you would need to know – weight and height limits, how to install the seat, how to clean the seat, etc. However, if you are unable to understand the information being provided through the manual, there are tons of great social media groups out there that offer more information. All you have to do is go onto the social media platform and search *"(insert your county's name) Car seat Safety"* for groups/pages. Please note that there *are* right and wrong ways to install a car seat so that it is safe and effective for your child. You can also (most likely) find local Child Passenger Safety Technicians (CPST) near you; to find one, just use a search engine and search *"local CPST near me."* These are trained experts regarding car seats, installation, and proper care. One piece of information that is not typically known by the general population, is that car seats need to be replaced when/if they are ever involved in a vehicular collision, big or small – even if it is only a little fender bender!!! However, stringing another piece of unknown information correlated with that, you should contact your vehicle insurance company to report the accident and that the car seat was involved. Insurance companies will replace the lost car seat. Speaking of replacing car seats… I would keep in the back of your mind, that car seats actually have expiration dates! That's right – check on the lower part of the car seat (as well as the base, if an infant seat) and there you will find an expiration date that the car seat is good until. If you go through a friend or marketplace kind of situation, always look out for those dates; however, please, *please* know that you never really know whether that seat has been involved in an accident or not, even if no damage is observed.

More Research…

Researching medical information when it pertains to anything related to your baby, should just be done immediately. Vaccinations are something that should be researched into, for sure. As I mentioned before, there are other places outside of the doctor where you can obtain more information. Each vaccination should have an insert that comes along with it. You can ask for a specific insert of any vaccine, or medication for that matter, from any pharmacy. Should you choose to vaccinate your baby, many pediatricians offer what's called a delayed scheduled; you can pick and choose how many shots that your baby receives at once. If there is anything that you take away from this section alone, please take away the term *vaccine injury*. They do exist; I have personal friends whose children have suffered with vaccine injuries, both physically and mentally. If you don't believe it for yourself, just… search it. See for yourself.

A Plug of Mucus… Excuse Me?

What the *actual fuck* is a mucus plug, you might be asking. To put it simply, it is a piece of mucus, but it is thick and it is to block the opening of your cervix. By blocking your cervix opening, the plug is able to keep out infections and bacteria. And guess what… it comes out. Unexpectedly, too! But, when you lose it, it can sometimes be an indicator that labor will start soon. However, just as with everything else, it differs for every woman;

you could go into labor within hours, or days, or even weeks after losing the mucus plug… it all depends on your body, really. Either way, the end is near! This is also usually when some providers will suggest getting a membrane sweep to kickstart labor (wait patiently – we talk about that soon!).

More Testing – This Time, From Your Lady Bits

Yes – you read that italicized font correctly – this testing will collect a sample (culture) around the vagina and rectum with a cotton swab. Let's start by explaining what exactly group B strep (GBS) is. GBS is a bacteria that lives in the body, that does not usually cause any serious illness[7]; only 1 or 2 babies out of 100 has been found born with GBS passed from Mom, if Mom was not treated with antibiotics during labor[7]. Should a pregnant woman test positive for GBS (or does not test at all) and somehow passed it along to the baby, the baby has potential to experience early-onset disease (within 12-48 hours after birth or up to the first 7 days), including meningitis, pneumonia, and/or sepsis[7]. Treatment usually involves antibiotics given intravenously once labor has begun. As with all medical testing/vaccinating, you can refuse it being done. However, you should know, that you *will* be pushed to receive antibiotics through an IV during birth if you decide not to test, and birth at a hospital.

Sweeping Those Membranes

So, if you are eager to kickstart labor and getting that baby out of you, a lot of women turn to membrane sweeps. Here is the thing to know first – *your cervix needs to be dilated in order to have this done.* I know, it sounds weird, right? What it is, is your provider using a gloved finger or two inserted into your cervix, sweeping across the membranes that amniotic sac to the uterine wall[8]. Essentially what this does is telling your body to release the chemicals that soften the cervix *(these chemicals are called prostaglandins, in case curiosity tends to kill your cat!)*. Do not go into a membrane sweep thinking that "this is it – my labor will start immediately after this gets done" – because honey, it does not… and it may never! These are not 100% certain to work for all women. If it does work, it could kick you into labor within hours, days, or even weeks. However, I will advise that this also begins your journey of self-advocacy during labor and delivery, regarding cervix checks. Again, getting a membrane sweep is entirely optional – even if your provider suggests it. And in my own personal opinion (along with probably dozens of midwives, doulas, and other natural-ish mamas), the less amount of foreign items going into your body when things are supposed to be coming out, the better. But – this method is actually only one method of inducing labor.

Induce Me!

I am not entirely sure if this has always been a "thing," but it feels like more recently, women have the option of being induced when they are near the end of their pregnancy. This scares me, only because the amount of knowledge and education (again) that women do not have on the matter, and what it does to their bodies, and their baby's body. I feel like after the stories that I have heard, and the research that I have done personally, I need to spread the information to pregnant women about being induced. It almost feels like women believe that it's some type of way of getting ahead of the curveball – like somehow being induced will allow you to avoid labor pains or the long, tedious labor of delivering a baby. I feel like it has become some type of cosmetic surgery that women are wanting to get their names on the wait list for! Now, do not get me wrong – there are actual legitimate medical reasons as to why a provider would suggest a woman be induced. However, lately, the reason that I'm hearing from women of being induced is because "my doctor says I can't go past 39/40 weeks." Well, I'm here to burst that bubble of yours, sweetie – your body was literally made to do this, and that baby will come whenever it is good and ready… and your body is good and ready. And that is the unsafe aspect of being induced – your body is being forced to push baby out, before your body is even prepared to get the job done. Ways of being induced include medication to soften and thin (also referred to as "efface"), and open/dilate your cervix. There is also the way in which your care provider ruptures your "break your water" by rupturing your amniotic sac, administering medicine that causes contractions, or utilizing a cervical ripening balloon. And yes, that last one is exactly what it sounds like: a balloon that they insert of your cervix, blow up, and let break your waters… crazy, right!?! All of these ways are fairly risky, because it is ultimately forcing your body to go into labor before its ready, but I am also here to touch on the medication that can be given for inducing labor, and the stuff that pregnant women need to know about it.

The medication that is used for induction is typically Pitocin®. I wish that there was a way to insert a link that you could just click on, because I would love to link the medication's own insert label! A simple internet search of "FDA Pitocin insert label" should get you exactly where you need to be. Find it, open it, read it for yourself. Learn!! On the fourth page of the insert, it blatantly lays out how "severe hypertension has been reported." Under the Adverse Reactions section of the insert label, you will read smaller reactions from being nauseous, to larger reactions like rupture of the uterus or anaphylactic reaction. Due to your body not yet being ready to birth a baby and it being given medication that forces the process, Mama will experience a labor that is much more difficult to manage. Why, you ask? Because in a normal labor, the uterine muscles get to relax in between contractions, however in an induced labor, the uterine muscle does not get that break, in turn causing stress on the uterus *and* the baby[11]. Also, Pitocin does not allow endorphins to be released in response to the increasingly stronger contractions, because the medication does not cross the blood-brain barrier[11]. And remember what I said earlier – about those special chemicals that women need to release during labor in order to successfully bring the baby down the cervix and out of our body? Endorphins was one of those chemicals! I would have to use at least two hands minimum to count the number of women I know that have been induced, for whatever the reason may have been, and had complications. Most of the women told me that the end result turned out to be an emergency C-Section. The biggest complaint that these women had in common was being hypertensive. Just remember – unless being induced is actually *medically necessary* for your and baby's health, just let your body continue to do the heavy lifting. Have faith in your body, and your baby!

chapter five
itssss baby time!

The pain that you feel in labor cannot be explained. All I can really say is, until you experience it, you won't really be able to describe it. Even after you experience it, you find trouble finding the words to describe it. The best way that I can describe it to you, is like someone was trying to rip my uterus and stomach out of my body with 7,000 knives. When labor begins, it starts off feeling like very strong period cramps that gradually get worse and worse. If you can imagine the absolute worst period cramps that you have ever felt in your entire life, multiple that feeling with fifteen. After a few hours of really, really strong cramps, you will get the urge to push the baby out. And before you ask how I know, or how your body will know, believe me – it just knows. Regardless of how you deliver your baby into this world, one thing remains true: our bodies were meant to procreate. That said, you should try to listen to your body. Labor is exactly that – *labor*! You and your body are working to get that baby out safely! The reason why your labor brings such excruciating pain is because while your cervix is opening for baby come out, the baby is also slowly being pushed down into the cervix. So, needless to say, there is a lot happening at one time. Not only does the physical stuff happen, but guess what else… Did you guess emotions? If so, you got it! Women release hormonal chemicals when they are giving birth – would you believe that!? *(Of course you would - we're superheroes. Duh.)* The chemicals released by women during childbirth are oxytocin ("the love hormone"), endorphins ("the pleasure hormone"), and adrenaline ("the fight or flight hormone"), and prolactin ("the mothering hormone")[12]. While giving birth, it truly does help your mental state – and in turn, your physical state – by being surrounded by people and things that make you feel love and happiness. Women that decide to give birth at home usually decorate an area that will be dedicated to where Mom will give birth; using fairy lights, or your favorite music, or being massaged all help increase those hormones and help guide you through the pain of labor. I remember having a playlist titled "Love" that I had my midwife play while I was laboring with my oldest; this playlist was chosen last minute, because I procrastinated literally until the last minute to make a birthing playlist. This playlist had almost all country love songs that I really enjoyed, but there were a few, umm, out of box tunes in there, too, that left my midwife and birth team questioning my choice in music! I thought that it was so hilarious – especially because it was not my intended playlist for the event! Needless to say – labor hurts like a bitch. But it is also true what you are told by other mothers… once the baby is born, you forget about the pain. Plus, there are so many options for pain management during childbirth to help you get through the pain!

Take This Damn Pain Away!

Thank goodness for pain management options that are available for women giving birth! I really do not know how a lot of women would have survived getting through labor and delivery had it not been for the meds that they were given to help ease the pain! Ever since I was little, I always recalled my mother telling me about the long needle that she had to get put into her spine while in labor with me just to help relieve some of the labor pain. I would always think to myself, *"oh hellllll no."* And, many years later, when it was my time to have children, I remembered that story… and my answer still remained the same! Luckily, the epidural is offered to all pregnant women, and for all of the pregnant women that can do needles like that, more kudos to you! Outside of epidurals, however, there are other types of pain management that is safe for Mom and baby. If you choose to go the *al naturale* way of childbirth, you will be taught a few different techniques through your birth classes that will seriously help get you through labor. I loved having the father of my children take his hands, put his palms together, and push down as hard as I wanted on my lower back. There are also techniques like bouncing on a birth ball, or moving your hips in the Figure 8 motion. I know that when I did not yet know that my labor had begun when I was having my oldest son, being in a really hot shower seemed to help; that is also a reason why baths are recommended for labor. And let me tell you from personal experience – having a birth pool filled with warm water and cute little lights to help set the ambiance really helped me get out of my head and body, and into a more serene place to allow my body and my mind to open in order to give birth to my baby. The water does something magical to you when you are in so much pain, trust my word.

Pain relief for women in labor has been around for as long as women have been having babies! I mean, I don't really know the *actual* date of when women began seeking pain relief methods during labor, but I imagine it was very early! At least as early of 1772, when Joseph Priestley discovered nitrous oxide and its pain-relieving properties[10].

Obviously, the type of pain management that birth centers/midwives are able to offer differ substantially when it comes in comparison to what hospitals are able to offer women in labor. There are two types of pain relief methods that hospitals typically utilize: analgesia, which is able to provide pain relief without any loss of muscle movement or feeling (does not stop pain completely); and anesthesia, which blocks most of the feeling as well as pain[9]. When it comes down to the actual types of pain relief offered, you have a few to choose from: systemic analgesia (opioids), nitrous oxide (laughing gas), local anesthesia (pudendal block), regional pain relief (epidural and spinal blocks), and general anesthesia[9]. Let's break it down to understand it a little bit better, shall we?

Systemic analgesia are opioids; the "systemic analgesia acts on the whole nervous system, rather than a specific area, to lessen pain.[9]" Don't worry – these won't knock you out entirely, but will probably have you feeling *really* mellow. If you have an IV hooked up, that is probably the way that you would receive the medication. On the flip side, as I mentioned that I only want to educate women on things that they do not have information on, I want to tell you about what could happen as potential side effects with choosing this form of pain relief. If you do not want to know, skim to the next few sentences – you are totally allowed! You should know that opioids have the tendency to lower your heart rate and breathing for a small bit of time – *along with baby's.* Because this medication is administered intravenously, it does enter into your baby's system; that said, your baby could come out a bit "out of it" as well.

Next up: good ol' laughing gas – nitrous oxide. To put into perspective, this is the stuff that dentists use when they are doing some teeth pulling or light work. You are usually given a mask to inhale the gas; you have total control over when and how much gas you inhale. But you should probably start inhaling at least thirty second before a contraction starts, just to ensure you are relieved of some pain. The gas is entirely odorless, and you are unable to taste anything in your mouth either. I have personally been given nitrous oxide by a dentist while pulling my two top wisdom teeth – and I will say, it did the job… although, I have no idea how it would help with the pain during labor and delivery. This was the method of pain relief that was discovered in 1772 by Joseph Preistley, and the pain-relieving properties had been first introduced to the public by Horace Wells, an American dentist, in 1844[10]. There have not been any adverse side effects identified, outside of feeling dizzy or nauseous while inhaling, however the feelings should go away within minutes.

Local anesthesia is usually what dentists also use, mostly when filling a cavity maybe. The anesthesia is injected into the body (in a woman delivering a baby's case, into the nerves that carry feeling into the vagina, vulva, and perineum[9]) with a needle. Utilizing local anesthesia is also referred to as a pudendal block. No safety risks have been identified from using anesthesia while giving birth, however there could be an allergic reaction or nerve/heart issues if the dose is too high.

What a lot of women are most common with, are epidurals – like my mother. An epidural can be administered shortly after labor has begun, and is inserted via a needle into your lower back, into your spine. Once the needle has been placed, a small, thin tube is inserted (needle removed) and left behind for the medication to be given as needed through the tube[9]. Pain relief should typically be felt within 10 to 20 minutes after the initial dose. Epidurals will usually allow you to stay awake, but lose most of the feeling into the lower-half of your body; a lot of women that have had epidurals have told me that there is a sensation to push, and there is pressure while pushing, but no pain. My mom will only talk about the needle, so there's that… But, as with all of the previous methods of pain relief, there are downfalls. Unfortunately, the amount of women that I personally know that have had epidurals have complained about a long-lasting back pain. Not only that, but there is the risk of missing the correct spot while administering the epidural; this was the scariest part about it to me, especially when my mother told me how she had to stay completely still while getting the epidural even though she was having contractions during the process!

Labor Tips and Tricks

You may be doubting yourself, and thinking *"There's no way that I can birth a baby the size of a damn watermelon!"* But you *can*! And very unfortunately for you… you *will!* No matter which way you bring your baby into this world, you *can* do it! And before you know it, it's over and you are staring into the eyes of the tiniest, most precious little soul. Well, I am about to blow your mind! I will share with you the things that my midwives taught me over the course of two natural births, and what I have learned from gathering my research and expanding my knowledge! Now, you really might think that I am totally off of my rocker with some of these ideas, but just trust me. You will come to learn that a lot of being pregnant, giving birth, and being a mother means giving up a lot of the control that you like to have!

1. *Intentional breathing.* This is the obvious one, right? Learning how to intentionally breathe. You can use prayers or guided meditations to help you find a rhythm to match your breathing to. What helped me was the 444 technique: breathe in for four seconds, hold your breath for four seconds, breathe out for four seconds, and then hold your breath one more time for four seconds.

2. *Take a shower/bath.* Like I said, that warm water is just so magical during labor.

3. *Birth ball.* This will help keep the baby aligned with your pelvis, making for a quicker trip down your cervix and into this world!

4. *Getting a massage.* Time to put your support partner to work! Have them massage you in your favorite places (preferably not the ones that got you into this spot to begin with!), and really try to melt away under their touch.

5. *Relax.* This goes hand-in-hand with getting a massage for the obvious reasons. Try to engage in anything that helps you relax, whether it be coloring or cooking, or just binging your favorite television series.

6. *Aromatherapy.* Although there has not been anything proven that aromatherapy proves pain relief, it does make people able to relax and release those special chemicals that we need during labor.

7. *Music.* Like I mentioned, I had a playlist that I used during my labor of my oldest. Again, even though it doesn't necessarily provide pain relief, it does cause pleasure!

8. *Keep it movin'.* Keep movin' and groovin'. The movement and pull of gravity will naturally bring the baby further down into the cervix, allowing for a much easier glide into this world!

9. *Visual imagery / Hypnobirthing.* Start thinking about your favorite people – your partner, your other children, whomever – at your favorite place, like maybe the beach or a special trip that you had or desire to go on. Try to allow yourself to go into a trance-like state. *(I highly, highly recommend looking on the internet for some hypnobirth videos, because this will be a blessing to use if you want to have an unmedicated birth!)*

10. *Hold ice*! Yup – hold ice in your hands for as long as you can! Or, another version of this, is holding a comb with the picks pressed into your fingers as long as a contraction. This will help distract your mind from one pain to another. *(This is also great to practice while you are pregnant, preparing for birth, because it will also teach you techniques to use to control your pain… like now!)*

Checking Your Cervix During Labor

So, we meet again, with the question of allowing foreign objects into our cervix when something is meant to be coming out. But this time, you are in labor, and more than likely have one thing on your mind: *get this fucking thing out of me!!* And if this isn't your first rodeo and you are reading this just for shits and giggles, you are probably getting a kick out of reading that, because you know the exact thoughts that I'm talking about! Anyway – you will be asked if you want to check how dilated your cervix is. How this is done, is by your provider sticking fingers up your lady bits and measuring the possible diameter of your cervix with said fingers. It doesn't sound great, does it? It's not – and it is extremely uncomfortable. Yes, I have had my cervix checked while in labor; I told you that I am nothing but honest and open with you. I had my midwife check my cervix while I was in labor with my oldest, because I was very eager for the pain to be over with; she checked me three times before I gave birth. Luckily, I had no consequences to deal with after the fact (like an infection). With my second, my midwife only checked me once; I asked her to check me about halfway through to see how far I had to go, and little to my surprise, she told the father of my children that I was ready to go, but told me that I was only "almost there!" *(Labor and delivery of my second son was much more painful and tedious for me, and she did not want to give me false hope in case it just did not happen right then.)* So, what should be the takeaway of this? Educate yourself. Learn about what could happen as a cause of cervix checks. Figure out what you would be comfortable with. And again, have a support partner or a doula that knows your birth plan and enforces it – make sure to include whether or not you would allow cervix checks and stand firmly on it. That rolls me right into my next subject…

Implementing Your Birth Plan

By this point, your birth plan should already be all done-up with the finishing touches on it, ready to go with you to the birth of your baby. Whatever you have on your birth plan, remember what I said earlier… as much as you may plan, birth will never go according to *your* plan; birth goes according to *baby* and *body*. But you do have control over a few things – like cervix checks! Also, other decisions to be made, like whether you want pain relief, what kind of pain relief you would be willing to get, fetal monitoring, what kind of position you prefer to birth in, and even saving the placenta. You can make it as simple as you'd like, with simply writing "Open to All Interventions" or customize it to your specific liking. The hardest thing about your birth plan, will be to actually get it implemented by your delivery team (if not a midwife and her team). In this case, this is where having a support partner and/or a doula comes in handy; this designated person will be the birth gatekeeper. Not that if the birth plan does not get implemented your way, the baby would not come out, because let's face it – that baby is coming out one way or another, whether anyone likes it or not. No, what I mean is that this person will be the voice for you while you focus on managing the pain from labor and safely delivering this baby earthside. I'm not saying that the hospital staff is *against* you in any way, but sometimes Mom's voice can be over-ruled or shaken in the moment, given the surrounding circumstances. We all already know that sometimes when we have to visit a doctor, we get spoken to in Doctor language and do not understand a lick of what was just told to us, then have to ask the nurse to translate it into a language we actually understand. So, to sometimes feel overpowered has been a commonly expressed emotion while giving birth at a hospital. *(Not for nothing, but this is typically where women are suggested to get a C-Section if "labor is taking too long," so just be sure to really know your body and the process of giving birth… or have an advocate by your side!)* Anyway… the time has come. Time to PUSH!

chapter six

the baby has arrived – now what?!

Congratulations!!! You did it!! The baby has safely arrived, and we have come to the other side of pregnancy! Now, you have entered the newborn phase of motherhood. And if you think pregnancy was a wild ride, I do not advise unbuckling for the next few… years. Your body is *still* changing! If you have decided to breastfeed, your body is changing by providing your baby with the proper nutrients; if you are not breastfeeding, your body is still changing inside! A woman's body takes time to heal properly; all of your organs and bones that were moved need to go back to where they came from! And, after the placenta comes out, you are left with a gaping hole the size of a dinner plate in your uterus that needs to heal completely!! So, let's go along the ride of navigating what to do after the baby has arrived, and what is in store for everyone!

After the Push

After the baby comes and you are finally done with all of that fu…. painful labor, and you have had the opportunity to hold and smell your new baby, you will prompted with more questions and decisions to make – unfortunately. Here is how the swing of things will go: baby's vitals will be checked, a physical will be conducted, measurements of weight, length, and head circumference will be taken, and vaccines will be offered. Within one hour of the baby being birthed, providers will offer the Vitamin K injection; this injection supposedly helps with blood coagulation *(providers will often say that if you birth a boy, this injection will help if you plan on getting him circumcised)*. Antibiotics are also going to be offered to be put into your baby's eyes to "help prevent infections." Again, here is *Mom's choice* of whether or not the baby gets the injection and eye drops. And again, here is where some providers will use their knowledge and education in a power play over new parents that have not done their research; you may be told that the state that you reside in requires

that your newborn get the injection and eye drops. But see, you –
we – are different. We are the ones that have done our research,
and we know whether or not our state of residence requires such
a thing. We *also* know that we can obtain an exemption form
from our local health department. I know that some of you are
going to ask *Why deny the injection and eye drops? Are they not meant
to protect my baby?* So, let's get into it…

WARNING – INTRAVENOUS AND INTRAMUSCULAR USE

Severe reactions, including fatalities, have occurred during and immediately after INTRAVENOUS injection of phytonadione, even when precautions have been taken to dilute the phytonadione and to avoid rapid infusion. Severe reactions, including fatalities, have also been reported following INTRAMUSCULAR administration. Typically these severe reactions have resembled hypersensitivity or anaphylaxis, including shock and cardiac and/or respiratory arrest. Some patients have exhibited these severe reactions on receiving phytonadione for the first time. Therefore the INTRAVENOUS and INTRAMUSCULAR routes should be restricted to those situations where the subcutaneous route is not feasible and the serious risk involved is considered justified.

CLOSE

I really only feel compelled to share the Boxed Warning
(otherwise known as the strongest warning that the FDA requires
if a medication's studies have a significant risk of serious/life-
threatening effects). So, here you go:

The First Few Days

Euphoria. Bliss. Perfection. Love. Safety. Fear. Sadness.
You will feel so many things during the first few days after having
your baby, let me tell you! You will probably go through every
emotion there is. You are in this twilight/honeymoon phase after
having a baby; your mind and body is high on endorphins and all
of those love chemicals, and you are able to hold the most perfect
little human ever created in your arms… and that perfect creation
is *all yours*. The first few days/weeks are a dream with your new
baby. It's kind of like the rest of the world melts away, and
nothing matters but you, that baby, and your partner. Time

vanishes, and your sleep schedule is literally run by that perfect little creation of yours. You also probably also have forgotten to shower or eat, because you do not want to miss a single thing that your new baby does. You will feel so full of love; but you may also feel fear and sadness. Why? For me, I was fearful that my baby was now on the outside of my body and I had to protect him in a whole new way, and from all new things; I felt a bit of sadness *because* my baby was no longer in my belly. Like I said – a full range of emotions. But it is totally okay, and nobody is judging you for any of it!! *(Just make sure to remember to shower once in a while…)*

Implementing Boundaries with Others

One of the more difficult challenges that I have heard that women faced after becoming a mother was being able to set ground rules with other people, and enforce them, specifically with family members. After you carry your baby for damn near ten months, and you are relishing in your reward of all of that hard work you did to ensure that baby was welcomed earthside healthy and safe, the last thing you want to do is let that baby out of your arms or sight. That baby is the equivalent of a golden egg in your eyes. Unfortunately, everyone else wants to see the golden nugget and relish in all its glory, too. The thing is, though, is that sometimes people let the excitement and urges get the best of them, and they can become pushy and persistent. I mentioned how my firstborn was born in June 2020 when COVID was still in its beginning phases and we still knew little to nothing about the illness – would you be shocked if I were to say that I still had family members pushing to come see the baby, and getting upset when they were not able to? Facts! First of all, I went into labor extremely unexpectedly one day, so the fact that the baby was coming the day that he came was a shock to even his mama. Secondly, I had an incredibly rough pregnancy with him, and I absolutely wanted to reap the benefits of my reward! And lastly, it was three months into COVID being worldwide spread, and I was petrified. I was not at all ready for anyone to come into my home with this unknown sickness causing people to die, or to share my new baby in general yet. I did not think to talk to family members before the baby was born *(mind you, I also thought that I had a few weeks before I had to!)*, so the ground rules were not set up and understood. The father of my children and I discussed what would happen if we had the baby at the hospital – who we would let come visit, what I preferred, etc. My partner and I were on two very different pages, because he wanted to invite a few family members of his, whereas I did not want anyone to visit until we were settled at home *(this discussion also took place pre-COVID, and before we had switched into the care of a midwife)*. After a few arguments with my partner and some family members' feelings being a little bit hurt, we made the decision to wait two weeks before allowing any family to visit at all. And, that's exactly what we did – the first family visitor that we had was my partner's father *(my mother was living with us at that time, so technically she was able to actually meet the baby first, though)*. It should be made important for you to set boundaries regarding the baby early on.

You will most definitely have to set boundaries when it comes to people giving your sweet new baby smooches, too. Since someone's lips are getting pressed against the baby's skin, they are transferring germs onto your baby – that should be common knowledge for anybody. Outside of just maintaining good hygiene in general, kisses can cause a few yucky issues that the baby could develop. There have been babies that have gotten RSV (Respiratory Syncytial Virus) that absolutely ruins a new baby's immune system and may even end up having the baby in the hospital on breathing assistance machines. Cold sores could also be passed along to the baby by kissing; I have seen pictures of a baby absolutely covered in cold sores after a family member kissed the baby's hand and the baby put her hand to her face –

and that baby was in the hospital because it had gotten so bad for her. Letting people smooch on your baby is *not* worth the risk; let them be upset with you. But again, do not just take my word for it – go do your own research, see the pictures and read the horror stories that families have wrote about their experiences for yourself.

Useful Crap to Have Near You

I am not sure if you, my lovely reader, is anything like me and use a nightstand, but if you do, I hope you are *not* like me in the sense of it always being full of junk! After having a baby, your nightstand becomes your go-to table, because you *should* be resting in bed with your baby for a few weeks after pushing that beautiful little creation out. Anyway, my issue was that I had no idea what I needed on my nightstand, and to keep on my nightstand, that would be useful for me and/or the baby. For instance, I am a Chapstick fanatic *(I literally have a car Chapstick, nightstand Chapstick, purse Chapstick, diaper bag Chapstick… I can go on and on)*, so I made sure to have a few back-ups available. I also made sure to keep a few high-protein snacks in my nightstand – and a few extra waters. It really all depends on what you feel as though you will need the most. There are women that keep their nipple cream on the nightstand after nursing, or women that keep the stuff to make a formula bottle there… it all depends on your needs, and the baby's needs. Pacis, burp cloths, an extra onesie on-hand, whatever.

Make Your Life Easier – Shit to Purchase ASAP!

In motherhood, you have to be clever. Sometimes you have to out-clever the kid. And if you think I am joking, I am not. Ask friends that are parents, they would probably agree with that statement. Finding things to make your life easier is just common sense. There have been so many great things invented for mothers to make their lives easier, it is insane! I don't even know where to begin, there are so many!

If you have not yet been introduced to the great world of baby carrying, let me gladly make the introduction. There are carriers, and wraps, and slings, and hip seats, *oh my!* First of all, you are going to need to try the different types of style on before making a sound decision. It would help a lot to ask your friends that you may know that baby carries; a lot of times, mothers know why they love their baby carrier and are eager to brag about it anyway! They are all different, though. Each one has its own good qualities, and you just have to find the one that best suits you. Chicco comprised a list of the six types of carriers: soft structured, wrap, sling, Mei-Tai, backpack, and hip seats[15]. Within the list, there are pros and cons to each type. Let me break them down for you:

1. Soft Structured Carriers: these are the types that probably comes to mind when you hear the words "baby carrier." They have two arm straps that buckle twice, a seat for the baby, and a waistband that buckles; all of the straps are adjustable and padded. This carrier can hold the baby in the front or the back. However, a lot of these carriers require an infant insert, because the baby is too small for the carrier.

2. Wraps: these are basically very long pieces of fabric, nothing else. There is nothing special about them (except maybe their beautiful designs), and it is all about how you tie the wrap that allows you to carry your baby. Wraps typically have a very long life to offer, and can be used from infancy to toddlerhood. You are able to wear the baby wherever you'd like – front, back, side – once you figure out how to properly and safely tie the wrap.

3. Baby Slings: (also referred to as ring slings) these are carriers, again, made of a piece of long fabric – but these have one ring at the end of each side of the fabric to fasten and carry your baby.

These carriers use the weight of the baby to keep the fabric from slipping out of the rings, so don't you fret – you won't drop your baby *(hopefully)*. This is another carrier that is difficult to maneuver, and some practicing might be involved.

4. Mei-Tai: these are your hybrid carriers, created by a combination of a soft-structured carrier and a wrap. There are long pieces of fabric that are tied around your body, but there is also two shoulder and waist straps to tie *(yes, tie)*. These carriers can also be used from infancy to toddlerhood and offer a long lifespan.

5. Backpack Carriers: these carriers were made for my outdoorsy mamas. These carriers were designed specifically to be worn on your bike, and often have two shoulder straps with buckles to fasten in the front. These carriers are super comfortable for the kiddos, but they are super bulky, so beware.

6. Hip Seats: these are essentially waistbands that have a cushioned seat for the baby with some side pockets. These carriers do not have shoulder straps, and were meant to help take majority of the weight off of your hip while carrying your child. These carriers probably should not be used for infants, however are great for toddlers.

I have to keep it real with you here – I bought a few different types of carriers! Unlike my advice to you that you are going to take, I did not take the time to go try any on to see what felt comfortable for me. *(Also, keep in mind that even if you do try on a carrier and find one that you think you will like, your opinion can totally change once the baby is here and in the carrier.)* I know for a fact that I had the soft structured carrier, sling, and a wrap. When both of my boys were fresh out of the womb, they both loved the wrap that I had (Baby K'Tan); they were no longer babies when they were inside of that thing – they were baby kangaroos. My oldest would have slept for eternity in that wrap if I would have let him!

That had to be my favorite, and most useful, baby item that I received. My second favorite would probably be the sling; it is super easy to use once you learn, and they have different fabric types that you can choose from. My sling was made of mesh, which I liked, living in Florida! Both of these carriers made life easier for me – I was able to secure them into their kangaroo pouch and go about doing what I needed to do, whether it was cleaning, cooking, laundry, or just soothing the kid. The soft structured carrier that I had for both of the boys was not bad, but they are definitely not made for infants, so unless you have the infant insert, you will find yourself waiting a little while before putting the baby in it safely. But once they are big enough, the carrier is great – it's simple to use, quick to throw on, and the baby likes it!

Here's the catch… Just like everything we have been talking about up until now, you need to do your own research on carriers before just throwing your infant into one. There are specific ways that the carrier should be sitting on you, and certain ways that the baby needs to be situated inside of the carrier. Here are some tips and tricks that are offered from the website, Happiest Baby[16]:

- Baby should be in the M-position while in the carrier
- Check the carrier's age and weight limits
- Make sure your carrier is snug, tight enough to have your baby lightly pressed to your body
- Mind what moves you make – always bend at the knees, not the waist
- Kissing Rule: your baby should be sitting high enough in the carrier for you to be able to lower your head and kiss their forehead
- Keep the baby's chin up at all times, and keep neck straight (should be able to fit one finger under their chin)
- If you plan on nursing in the carrier, learn how to nurse safely

- T.I.C.K.S. Rule:
    o Tight: carrier should be tight with baby high, upright, and head supported
    o In view, always: baby's face should always be visible when you look down
    o Close enough to smooch: baby should be high enough to be able to lean down to kiss on the head
    o Keep baby's chin off their chest: do not let their chin fall onto their chest, restricting breathing
    o Supported back: baby's back should be in a natural shaped position, and your hand should always be placed on the baby for support while bending

The next purchase that will make your life as a mother a little bit easier would be an infant chair. And I'm not talking about highchairs or boppy pillows. I would probably refer to them as baby *loungers*. These are the chairs that your baby is able to essentially lay in. What makes them so great is that you can move the seat to wherever you are in the house – in the kitchen cooking, taking a quick shower – and the baby can chill while they are in your direct line of vision! My oldest son practically lived in his, he loved it so much. The best part was how I was able to actually shower after having a newborn, thanks to this chair! As far as a boppy is concerned, there have actually been *"voluntary"* recalls on them, after babies have suffocated while asleep[17]. One pillow that would more than likely be useful for Mom is a nursing pillow. Nursing pillows are typically semi-circle pillows that you either just place around your torso while nursing, or can fasten buckles connected to straps on the pillow while nursing. Having a swing is also an advantage, because it will help lull the baby to sleep and/or keep them entertained for a little while so that you can get some shit done! A lot of parents will also turn to the sit-me-up seats. And again, those are something that you should do some research on before deciding to purchase. Why? Same reason as the carriers – your baby's hips have to be factored in. These seats can be great when your baby is old enough to keep their head and neck straight and possibly sitting up, but you should also be warned that the chairs are not as supportive as you may think. Because the baby's torso isn't supported, specifically the ribcage, the baby would need to use core muscles… but, they probably do not know how to use those yet. If you do end up purchasing/being gifted one of these seats, I would recommend only keeping the baby in it for a few minutes opposed to longer. Again, do your own research to draw your own conclusions on any products that you are thinking about purchasing… I know that I don't only take others' words for it – I need the facts to back it up!

Baby's First Pediatrician Appointment

One of the first things on your To Do list for the baby is to schedule the first appointment with the pediatrician of your choosing. Remember how you had started gathering information for pediatricians earlier? Now is the time for you to use that information. Before scheduling the baby's first pediatrician appointment, though, there is one very important task that you must complete first: report the baby's birth to your insurance company (even Medicaid). By reporting the baby's birth, it should kickstart the baby's insurance (or will soon). After that, go ahead and call the pediatrician office to schedule the first appointment. At the first appointment, make sure to be prepared to fill out a shit ton of paperwork; make sure to have as much family history on Mom's and Dad's side of the family. In the room, the pediatrician will give your baby a look-over, ensuring that everything is there and intact in the places it should be. The pediatrician will also check the baby's reflexes, measure the baby, and offer any guidance or recommendations pertaining to the baby's weight and feeding. The pediatrician might also ask some postpartum questions for Mom, checking for any postpartum mood disorders or concerns. Also, vaccinations may be discussed, as the baby will be due to get the first round of vaccines; this is where all of the research that you have done on vaccines come in hand in order for you to make an educated decision. Should you have a male baby, and you have made the decision to circumcise, this is the visit to ask the pediatrician for any pediatric urologist recommendations/referrals for the surgery.

Spoil the Baby – But Spoil Mom More

Having a new baby around can be so exciting for everyone – it's a brand-new baby to dote on! Who wouldn't be excited!? But here's the thing to remember… Mom just pushed out a baby the size of a watermelon out of a teeny tiny hole. She is going to need time to heal and recover – both physically and emotionally. Even if Mom isn't experiencing a postpartum mood disorder, she will need some emotional support. Speaking from experience, being able to grow a baby inside of you is magical and all, but you know that the baby is safe (for the most part) inside of you… and when the baby is actually here in your arms, your emotions start flying because now the baby is on the outside of you and it's a whole new world for both of you. Also, Mom doesn't just become Mom overnight; try to remember that "mother" is only a title – not the person. While Mom is physically recovering, expect to do most of the heavy lifting for a while if you are a partner/spouse; take the household chores by the neck and get them done, take care of the baby as often as you can, or even just make sure that the house doesn't crumble with the touch of a woman for a few weeks. To best mentally support the new mama, try to check in as often as you can with her; ask her how she's feeling, but also give her the space that she needs to make the transition into becoming a mother. Be empathetic towards her – her emotions are going to be literally all over the place still for a little while longer. If the decision has been made to breastfeed (or not), support Mom's decisions to the best of your capabilities. If there are friends or family members wanting to push themselves into the hospital/house to see the new baby and Mom isn't ready, listen to her. *Listen to her.* Advocate for her. Support her. Love her. And when she is back on her feet doing the damn thing again, make sure that you remind her every chance you get that she is Superwoman and you are and that baby are so blessed to have her as Mom and partner. I know that it may sound super cheesy, but Mom's mental health heavily relies on the support around her, physical and emotional. Without having that support, she could easily develop a postpartum mood disorder.

chapter seven

after baby arrives: your new life

Just like pregnancy, women have to deal with the everchanging emotional rollercoaster in postpartum, too. Yuck – I know. A woman's mental health after she gives birth is so, so important. Hormones are still absolutely raging through your body, and even more so now that the baby is actually here in your arms and you get to stare at him/her without ever glancing away. You will feel like you are in this mix of being in the honeymoon phase and being in a fog so thick that you can hardly see. The days go by so slowly and fast all at the same time, and you have no idea what day it is or when the last time you showered was. You are stuck in a new world of being a mom, learning how to nurse/feed your baby, learning your baby and their mannerisms to the best of ability (which, do you ever?), and just trying to keep your head afloat somehow. And if you are in a partnership after having a baby, there are even new and different emotions wrapped around that person and relationship. It is a *lot* to navigate. A lot of feelings. So, making sure that Mom's mental health is okay should be a top priority – for everyone. Because the reality of it is, if Mom is not okay, she is not caring for herself or for her baby to the best of her abilities. Loved ones should keep up with the mama; be sure to check in with her, drop off pre-made dinners, leave coffee at her doorstep, offer to come over and clean the house… Most importantly, be aware of signs to look out for in new mothers, and know the new mama in your life well enough to know when/if she is off.

Learning the things to look out for is the most useful thing that you could do as a new mother, or as someone that has a new mother in their life. For instance, there are three main types of postpartum mood disorders: (1) baby blues, (2) postpartum depression, and (3) postpartum psychosis. Now, these two mood disorders are very different from one another, although may sometimes have similar symptoms. Symptoms for both of these disorders include feeling sad, experiencing crying spells, loss of appetite, and having trouble sleeping. However, these symptoms only last for about two weeks after the baby is born, whereas postpartum depression lasts much longer. Other symptoms for postpartum depression include feelings of harming oneself and/or the baby, feeling as though you cannot connect to/bond with the baby, having memory and attention problems, or having feelings of guilt, worthlessness, or like you are a bad parent[12]. Symptoms of postpartum depression are more severe than those of the baby blues, and last for a much more extended amount of time. Topping postpartum depression in the severity of symptoms, postpartum psychosis is another mood disorder to make sure to watch out for. Symptoms of this disorder typically beginning developing within one week after giving birth, and includes symptoms like feeling confused or lost, paranoia, obsessive thoughts about the baby, sleep problems, excessive energy, hallucinations, and thoughts of harming oneself or the baby[14]. A lot of factors can go into why a woman may experience any one of these mood disorders, but having a history of depression or issues with your partner, for instance, could contribute to women getting it. Should you (or someone you love) experience any of these mood disorders, you should look into locating local support groups (again, a simple internet search will suffice). Also, be sure to tell your doctor (whether it is your primary care physician, your OB, or your midwife) and seek professional mental health help.

Oh Shit… Who Am I Now?

Becoming a mother is… something. I do not even have the words to describe it, that's how insane it is! One minute, you are just you… the next, you are you, plus a smaller you. And you will never be just you again. Does that make sense? But again, "mother" is just a title, not the person. Although, some women (myself included) have trouble with this transition, and go through a bit of an identity crisis. After having my firstborn, I remembered being in a constant fog; I felt like I had no idea what day it was, time did not exist, life did not go on outside of the walls of me and the baby. And then I realized, that life *was* going on outside of the walls – without me now. I obviously just had a baby, so I was on maternity leave from my job, the father of my children went back to work a few days after having our son, and my mother that lived with us at the time continued going to work during the weekdays. So, I was left home all alone – just me and this new tiny human that I was responsible for. I was barely sleeping, which made things *a shit ton* times harder than they really were. And, again, if you just so happen to be a parent already and you are reading this, you know that sleep deprivation shit that I am talking about! It was like my whole life that existed pre-baby had somehow disappeared right before my very own eyes, and now my sole purpose was to care for this tiny human. *WHAT!?* When the baby cried, I was the one that comforted him; when the baby was hungry, I was nursing and was the only one that could feed him at the time; when the baby was tired, I was the parent that rocked him to sleep. It seriously felt like my entire being was just a vessel to be used up by this tiny human. And I had no idea how to feel about that, or how to properly navigate the transition into motherhood. And by no means am I saying that my mother was unsupportive of me and/or me transitioning into a mother, but unless someone goes through something similar (or you're a trained professional), they have no way of knowing how to help and best support you. Like I mentioned, having that support is so, so needed for Mom during this time. A lot of the stories that I have heard from women that fell into postpartum depression had a lot to do with losing who they were before the baby and having difficulty coming to terms with who they became after the baby. So, with that I will say *(for the umpteenth time)*, "Mother" is only a title, not the person.

The best piece of advice that I can give to you if you are

having these same feelings, is: 1, seek professional help; and 2, don't let your new title consume you. Yes, life might be different after having a baby – you will probably lose a few friends, family relationships/dynamics might be strained, you may not have much of a social life anymore, finances may be stressed about, you might end up being a full-time stay-at-home mother – but learn how to ride the waves. There are going to be times when your cute little baby will be up every hour on the hour for nights in a row, so believe me when I say, you just have to find things that work best for you, your baby, and your new way of life. Motherhood – parenthood – is like a dance; we are all learning how to go as it comes to us. There have been so many parents out there that have led adventurous lifestyles (like full-time travelers, for example) that have had children, and instead of changing their lives entirely, they made room for the baby in the lives that already existed. What worked for the family of full-time travelers was bringing their baby along with them on their adventures; the baby meshed into the lifestyle that already existed. On the opposite hand, you have families that *have* completely changed their lives for their baby – maybe that same full-time traveling family ended up settling in a quaint little town until the baby gets old enough for them to be comfortable enough to bring the child on their travel adventures. My point is: your birthed the baby *into* your family, so allow what meshes the baby into your family to work in the best ways to allow an easier transition.

Paternal Postpartum Depression

Although paternal postpartum depression is not a universally accepted diagnosis, it can be clinically diagnosed using the DSM-5 criteria[18]. Men experience similar symptoms of PPD that women often display: irritability, indecisiveness, and emotional blunting. Communication in your relationship with your partner is going to be the biggest thing to improve in your relationship after the baby is born; emotions should be discussed, and mental health checks should be done regularly on one another. Men are less likely to express their emotions like women, however if a man begins displaying similar symptoms in which you would find a woman with diagnosed with PPD, he should seek professional help. It is no unknown fact that men do not enjoy talking about their feelings *(okay, most of them do not at least)*, so being aware of what to look out for will be the more useful in this situation. If the man begins to lose interest in things that they once enjoyed doing, begins heavily drinking/using recreational drugs, or no longer wants to engage with others, these could also be symptoms being displayed.

Men also have this stigma around fatherhood that there are certain expectations to meet as a father. For example, fathers are believed to be macho and not emotional. There is this stigma around fatherhood and how men should act in fatherhood, and it is so unhealthy for men as fathers! There is this stigma that men are just the work horses – they go to work to provide for their family and that is the sole purpose of their existence as a father now. The emotional and mental load that fathers carry is actually a lot more than we think or realize. Because fathers are usually the primary providers of the household, they lose time with their baby because they have to go to work. If they don't go to work, they don't make the money and can't provide. So, to sum up this section – men can experience postpartum depression just like women can. Be kind and easy on the daddies, too.

Romance After Baby

Relationships are already difficult without babies involved… but after having a baby, especially your first baby, expect some rocky areas ahead in your relationship. Having a baby changes a lot of things, including relationships… and sex. There have been actual books published giving women advice on

how to not hate your partner after a baby! The father of my
children and I went through a pretty rough patch after each of our
sons were born, if I'm being totally honest here. But it has been
said by generations before us, that parenting is fucking hard. And
typically, the stages from infancy to elementary-aged is the
timeframe where couples have the most challenging times in their
relationship. If you were having troubles in the relationship
before the baby came along, I would highly advise not to expect
the baby to change anything. Because let's be real – even the
strongest of the couples go through issues after having a baby.
There are different stressors now, and I'm not talking only the
new baby to care for; I'm talking about new financial stress,
emotional stress, mental stress, physical stress, etc. etc. So, it is no
wonder that relationships are strained! It is all in how you
navigate the new titles ("Mom" and "Dad") and the new
stressors that will matter and get you a positive outcome for the
relationship. If you begin having issues that seem to be much
larger than you are able to fix, and you want the relationship to
last, it could also be beneficial into looking into couples
counseling. The biggest hurdle that I faced with my partner after
having our oldest was communication; I was not expressing my
needs to him, and so my needs were being unmet. It took a lot of
time to navigate how to care for my baby, care for myself as a
new mother, and care for my relationship and partner. It is a
complete juggling act – but it is a juggling act that you should not
be juggling alone. Sex may even be a bit different after birthing a
baby vaginally. First of all, sex should be avoided for the first six
weeks at absolute minimum to allow Mom's body to heal
properly. Secondly, sex is going to feel funny for the first time
after giving birth. Things will feel out of place, or different than
they did before… Keep in mind that you just gave birth to a
whole ass human, and it is going to take some time for things to
be back to normal – if they ever go back to normal. And I
definitely do not want to scare you by saying that, but I mean,

would you expect everything to go back to how it was before the watermelon-sized baby came out of you!? Be patient. Be kind to yourself. Be gentle. And use protection, because girl, you are the most fertile after having a baby – so if you aren't planning another one immediately and don't want Irish Twins, wrap that willy!

Ain't No Shame Like Mom Shame

Mom-shaming is real, y'all. And don't be surprised when you experience it for the first time. Everyone – and I mean everyone – judges mothers. You will be judged if you stay at home full-time with your baby and not work; you will be judged if your baby goes to daycare or a babysitter while you work. You will be judged for the clothes that your baby wears, or what type of stroller you are pushing around. You will be judged for the clothes that you wear, too. You will be judged on whether or not you vaccinate your children, or decide to formula feed versus breastfeed. If you do not already, it is high time to develop some thick skin! There are so many types of mothers out there – from the types that allow their children screen time, to the ones that don't. My advice to you about this is to just keep your mouth shut. At least until you get a good feel for the other person's vibes. And also, only if you are comfortable with divulging any type of information about you, your kid, or your parenting preferences. Be mindful of judging others yourself too, though. And should you ever run into being judged by anyone at all, take it with a grain of salt and go about your business.

Another thing that you should probably get used to, is people giving you unsolicited parenting advice. Let me tell you – people have no shame at all when it comes to this, either! There have been women that have been approached by literal strangers in public being given unsolicited advice about what-the-hell-ever having to do with their child. *The audacity!* Whether it's strangers, family members, friends, or other mothers that you meet, you will more than likely hear quite a bit of unsolicited advice throughout your pregnancy, and motherhood. The biggest lesson that I had to learn when it came to unsolicited advice when I wanted to let my mouth open to others, was that 1, I hate it when it's done to me, and 2, if it's not hurting me, my kids, them, or their kids, why does it matter to me? Who cares what kind of food is given to someone else's kid? Who cares if a mother decides to only dress their kid in organic cotton or not? If it's not you or your family, then it should not matter one ounce to you.

Daycares – Pros, Cons, and Assistance

If you are a mother that has chosen to place their baby into a daycare, chances are, you are already a little bit of an emotional blob. So, let me try to help as much as I can with this one. First of all, daycares are full to the brim, majority of the time! That said, you will have to spend a lot of time doing some research and making calls to see if a daycare has availability, or when they may. Now, the most useful answer here will be *when* you want the baby to start daycare; if you are pregnant and have to get back to work by a specific date, I would begin calling and doing your research while you are still pregnant. That way, you can put your baby on the wait list and it be your baby's turn to fill a spot by the time your date to return to work rolls around. After doing some research, make to physically go to these daycares to tour them. You are going to want to get inside of them, go on a full tour, meet staff members, see other children and how they are interacting within the environment, and generally get a feel as to how you feel about the daycare. Most importantly, talk about the prices. The weekly fee for a newborn baby is going to be drastically different than the weekly price of a potty-trained three-year-old. The price difference could also vary when it comes to a standard daycare facility versus an in-home daycare. *(If you are choosing to go with a nanny or babysitter, please just make sure to do your due diligence and get references and a background check for anybody that will be around your baby!)*

With daycare, there are pros and cons – just like with literally everything else. A lot of mothers aren't comfortable with daycares, and often seek in-home daycares for their needs. Regardless, there will be other children around. That said, the pros will be: your child develops socialization skills; your child will be in a learning environment; the parents will be able to successfully work without having to worry about their child; and *(hopefully)* your child is being well taken care of while they are in daycare. On the flip side, there are the cons as well: daycares are cesspools for germs; your child will more than likely pick up a few not-so-great habits; and you do unfortunately lose time with your baby. Your needs and lifestyle will ultimately impact your decision on whether or not daycare would be suitable for you and your family.

Now, let me tell you a little secret… If you do choose to go down the standard daycare facility route, there are assistance programs that exist to help parents (especially single parents) afford daycare. Reverting back to that simple internet search again – doing a quick little search will probably get you the information that you need. But just being aware that there is help available is the first step.

The Controversial Topic of Sleep Training

One topic that has been pretty controversial in the parenting world is that of sleep training a child. There are so many opinions surrounding sleep training. And, go figure, there are a few different methods that you could try – or not try. Technically, there are five main methods that you have the option of choosing from. Let's break it down:

1. The Ferber Method. People often refer to this method as the "graduated extinction" method. This method is named after the doctor that developed it. Essentially, parents set time intervals to go back and check in on the baby after the baby is laid down, however should not to pick the baby up from the crib; these intervals can be done in five minutes, ten minutes, fifteen minutes, etc. Parents can use patting or lowly talking to the baby until the baby is quieted before resetting the time interval to repeat the process.

2. The Chair Method. This method includes parents keeping a chair right next to the baby's crib. The parent would put the baby to bed, sit in the chair, and not leave the bedroom until the baby is asleep. When the baby falls asleep, the parent would leave the room; if the baby were to wake up while you're trying to escape the room, you would just go sit back in the chair until the baby was back asleep. And with every night, the chair would get moved further and further away from the crib, until the chair is no longer in the room.

3. The Fading Method. Basically, you take what you typically do to get your baby to sleep and as each night passes, the time doing it would decrease more and more. Whether you use rocking, babywearing, or doing cartwheels to put your baby to sleep – it doesn't matter, only the time matters.

4. The Pick-Up/Put-Down Method. If you put your baby to bed, and they begin fussing, you should try to let it happen for a few minutes before going back into the bedroom and picking the baby up to get soothed. Once the baby is calm in your arms, try to put the baby back down in the crib before they have completely fallen asleep in your arms. And if they

start to fuss again… repeat the process again and again until the baby is out for the night!

5. The Cry-It-Out Method. This is probably the most talked-about method in the world of parenting – and if you choose to do this method and discuss it, just be prepared to have opinions expressed. Once the baby has gone through the normal bedtime routine and placed into the crib, you would leave. Period. You would leave the baby in the crib until they fall asleep, whether they fall asleep by screaming or laughing.

The method that you choose should be what you believe to be best for you and your baby. And do not fret – if you feel like you have chosen a sleep training method that does not seem to work for you or the baby, you can most definitely switch methods. Your own parenting style and personality should be taken into consideration when choosing a sleep training method. Why? Because you don't want to choose a method that conflicts against who you are as a person, or how you want to parent your child. Again, if you start with a method and end up liking it for whatever reason, you have the freedom to change the method. Just remember that, along with any other parenting feat, sleep training will be emotionally and sometimes physically draining for the parents too, no matter the chosen method. Sleep training takes time; think about training a puppy… it's basically the same thing, without hair and a shorter tongue!

When it comes to sleep training, the one thing that they don't warn you about, are the sleep regressions. Yes, there are regressions! What exactly does that mean, you ask? Say that you just spent all of this time getting the baby sleep trained, right… now, they are able to sleep well and hopefully through the night. A sleep regression is the big wrench that gets thrown into your perfectly pieced-together sleeping masterpiece; a sleep regression will cause the baby to either have trouble falling asleep or staying asleep. Although sleep regressions can really happen at any age, they usually occur while your baby is going through and/or reaching developmental milestones. So, just revert back to the method that you started sleep training using, and stick to your guns! Sleep regressions *will absolutely* feel like you are dying a slow death if you allow them to!

chapter eight
the first two years

During the first two years, you will experience so much with your baby! I highly recommend taking monthly milestone pictures from 0 to 12 months – although your picture gallery will already be super full of baby pictures, too! You get to watch your baby's face start off being this tiny, smooshy newborn face to this little face that holds its own features and personality! It's fucking awesome and sad at the same time, because time absolutely does fly by right before your eyes. You will go from being fascinated that your baby reaches for toys, to padding your furniture because they are trying to fly off of it. But before you get there, and before you are able to swallow the fact that everything happens exactly when it is supposed to happen (including baby milestones), you will probably question if your baby is "on track" a lot. Try not to compare your baby to other babies. The perfect example is my second born; he is growing up with an older brother showing him the ropes, and could be perceived as more developed than another baby the same age. There is no perfect science behind when your baby *will* reach the developmental milestones, but they *should* be somewhere in the same timeframe as other babies the same age as yours.

By three months old, your baby should develop physical skills, such as raising its head, opening/shutting hands, grasping onto toys, and bringing hand to mouth. Developed social skills would include the baby smiling at people, playing with people and imitating some movements and/or expressions. Your baby should also be recognizing familiar faces and objects from a short distance, using hands and eyes in coordination, and following objects as they move. From four months to seven months old, your baby should be rolling over from both sides, sitting unsupported, holding weight on legs, social playing, responding to emotional expressions, exploring things with their hands and mouth, watching themselves in the mirror, and transferring objects from one hand to another. And, from eight months to twelve months, your baby should be crawling forward, pulling up to stand, walking while holding onto furniture, crying when parents leave, preferring certain people/objects, finger-feeding self, and imitating gestures. Your baby will also begin to use items in the correct way, and even finding hidden objects! And, just to make sure that I properly prepare you – your baby *could* start walking before the age of one!

After your baby turns one is when things start getting exciting. And I find myself saying, again – buckle up, honey. Your baby will start following simple commands, pointing at things that pique their interest wanting to show you, and may even begin to enjoy pretending during playtime. This is also the age where you are able to ask your baby to go retrieve something, and they should be able to go into the other room to get an object and bring it back! *(See – I told you – exactly like training a puppy!)* Your baby is becoming a toddler now, and it feels unreal hearing your baby's little voice forming sentences and speaking to you! Fun fact: your child typically picks up about one new word per week between 18 months to 24 months old! By the age of two, your *toddler* should be able to speak multiple two-word sentences and/or phrases, have a vocabulary established of 50-100 words, be (mostly) understood by adults, and be able to follow one-step commands without using gestures.

Emotional intelligence also begins developing at a very young age for your baby. As early as your baby being born, they exhibit two emotional responses, which include attraction and withdrawawl[19]; babies are able to show attraction to things that pleases, comforts, or stimulates them, as well as withdraw from any unpleasant stimulation, such as physical discomfort[19]. *(Social smiling is actually a sign of your baby developing emotional intelligence!)* By the time your baby is around the age of six to fifteen months, they begin to develop separation anxiety and stranger wariness (aka, afraid to be in the presence of strangers). This is also when your small one will begin utilizing physical self-soothing strategies, like sucking their thumb or getting attached to a "stuffie." Your child will begin picking up emotional ques from others as well, especially their parents; they will even look at others to clarify how to respond to situations that they are unsure of. Unfortunately, this is when the term "emotional self-regulation" comes into play. Self-regulating has been one of the biggest hurdles to me as a parent, especially to a toddler. It is put into our hands to teach our babies how to be able to regulate themselves appropriately whenever in a heightened emotional state. For example, if your child sees you react in anger to small things, they absorb that into their little minds, and think that anger is the appropriate response to situations. Now, you are probably thinking to yourself that it doesn't sound so hard or bad, but the truth is, when you are triggered by something, you may not necessarily stop to think about how you react or respond and ultimately show an inappropriate emotional response to the trigger. Being able to understand your triggers and regulate yourself is the best thing that you can learn and try to do in the moment when it comes to this point in parenting. And believe me, the process is not always pretty. For instance, I *cannot stand* the high-pitch pterodactyl screaming that my son does; I have had to ask myself *why* so often, and stop myself from wanting to shove a rag into his mouth to make him stop screeching! You will definitely learn a lot about yourself while parenting and raising kids. The next hurdle would be the fact that your kiddo has literally no idea how to self-regulate or manage emotions… so, you are often just left picking up the pieces of a meltdown that just ensued, wondering how the hell you are going to survive this stage with your sanity intact *(update: still questioning that)*. As a parent, it is all left in our hands; you can teach your baby that whenever they become angry, it is okay to walk away and scream into a pillow or turn to violence. Just remember – what you teach them will stay with them into adulthood, and who they become as an individual… and most importantly, how they will treat others.

Pesky Little Phases

It is not an uncommon fact that every child goes through phases throughout their adolescence. Obviously, every child will be different (as they are with everything else) in terms of how much they lean into the phase. And what I mean by that, is how much the kid engages in the phase – like biting. Will the child be a biter, or will the child not really engage in biting at all? But typically, every child goes through a phase or two… or ten. These behaviors usually involve biting, hitting, and screaming. Essentially, it can all be led back to the developmental milestones; a child will typically begin biting things when they start exploring their mouth, as early as six months old. Teething could also be a factor into why a child began to bite others. Or perhaps your child has taken to biting as a way of expressing themselves. Once your child hits the age around two years old, it would not be unlikely that the child begins to bite or hit as a way of expressing frustration. If your child attends some type of daycare or is around other children that hit or bite, they could also pick up those pesky behaviors from their peers. The best thing that you could probably do whenever your child has seemed to have picked up one of those pesky behaviors, is to just go with the flow the best that you can. Do not take it to heart, because it is something that just about every parent has experienced at one point or another. Be persistent in reinforcing good behavior (you know, the opposite of the current behavior), and try to stay patient.

The "Terrible Twos" and…. More Mom Guilt

As your once-very-small baby grows older and bigger, you begin experiencing a whole new type of Mom Guilt. For me, it had a lot to do with if I was doing this whole mom thing correctly. When my oldest hit eighteen months old, it was like this tiny demon that would get pissed off if you looked in his direction possessed his body and my once sweet little baby boy was this demanding, temperamental little crotch gremlin. I questioned what I did wrong, or if I was just ruining him by doing/not doing things. I questioned if I was spending enough time with him, wondering if I "babied" him too much... I questioned literally everything. It was like I had no idea who my son was, and had to relearn him entirely all over again, as I had to do when he was a fresh little newborn nugget. And it's funny, because I am going through the very aggressive toddlerhood era with my oldest as I write this, and I had recently met a mother whose son had just turned one a few months earlier, and she was doting on and on about how her son is the sweetest baby; I ended up telling her to wait until he turns eighteen months and report back to me. It isn't that they turn "terrible" when they are close to two years old – it's just that they are learning that they have emotions and again, are unable to regulate those emotions. These tiny humans only know how to react the way that they have gotten their needs met so many times before – screaming or crying, typically. But now, the screaming and crying has turned into tantrums. And quite frankly, they are what I would call as purely explosive. Not only that, but your baby is in that weird in-between stage of still having to rely on adults but also wanting to be more independent. "No" becomes a well-known word, for both you and your baby. Although I tried my best at *not* saying the word no to my toddler, my attempts landed on deaf ears it seemed... and when your toddler is using your couch as his personal trampoline with only the tile floor to catch his fall, the quickest go-to became the word no. On the flip side, this is where my son also began to tell *me* no when he was instructed or asked to do things that I guess he just did not want to do at the moment. Let me tell you – toddlers truly test your inner gangster.

Like I said, motherhood has been *the* most humbling experience for me. And quite frankly, if motherhood *(parenthood, really)* doesn't humble you in the slightest, I would highly recommend looking very closely in the mirror and asking yourself why not… because we all have spots that could use some shinin', darling. And that brings me straight to my next point…

"Gentle" Parenting – and "Non-Gentle" Parenting

I am sure that in no time, there will be some other, more advanced type of parenting that comes along and is referenced in days to come, but right now, there is the parenting style that is referred to as "gentle parenting" that's big. Let me start by prefacing with this: when I grew up, I got spanked when I was bad. I got grounded – from toys, from friends, from going out, from driving, from going to school dances… and when I was really bad, I got spanked on my butt by a belt. I have even gotten a smack to the face a time or few for back-talking. So, when I tell you that gentle parenting is everything *opposite* of all of that, that is the best way that I can describe it to someone. But I will also say this – gentle parenting is leaning towards a way of breaking generational curses that have been needing to be broken. Gentle parenting is a style in which parents use respect, boundaries, empathy, and understanding to allow the child to work with the parent in expressing feelings in an acceptable manner[20]. A lot of people have a misconstrued conception about gentle parenting, typically thinking that it's the parents allowing their child to get away with murder without any type of disciplinary actions… but it is not. Those generational curses that I mentioned have only done one thing successfully: create generations worth of emotionally immature, broken adults. *(And this is absolutely to not fault of our own, because our parents didn't know any better at the time… but now we do!)* Gentle parenting focuses on teaching your child that it is okay be frustrated, but it is not okay to scream at the top of your lungs when you feel frustrated. Gentle parenting helps teach the child that it's okay to have emotions, and express emotions, but doing so in a healthy, beneficial manner. There have been studies that suggest that gentle parenting and encouragement could decrease the risk of anxiety in kids, as well[20].

As mentioned, gentle parenting is only one type of parenting style that exists. There are plenty types of others. And just like with anything else pertaining to parenting and raising babies, you have to pick and choose which style works best for you and your family. Again, you have the freedom of choice to do whatever you want! Other parenting styles include: permissive, authoritarian, authoritative, and uninvolved. Without going into much specifics about each one individually, I will give you a quick rundown:

- Permissive
  - Rules exist but not enforced
  - No consequences
  - "Kids will be kids"
- Authoritarian
  - It's your house, your rules
  - Child's feelings do not matter
  - "Be seen, not heard"
- Authoritative
  - Effort into having a positive parent/child relationship
  - Reasons given behind rules
  - Set limits, enforce rules, give consequences, and feelings are considered

- Uninvolved

- o Don't ask questions about child's day/life
- o Don't know where your child is or who they are with
- o Don't spend a lot of quality time with child

As always, my suggestion to you would be to do your own research. Luckily for you, the chosen parenting style does not have to be permanent if it doesn't feel comfortable for you. I will say, though – try to keep in mind that the parenting style that you do end up choosing and implementing, will have the most effect on the adult that your baby will grow up to be.

chapter nine

the [uncensored] expectations of motherhood

I know that I said that I would keep my personal opinions out of this book, but I may have told a tiny white lie about that. I mean, I feel like I was pretty successful in keeping my personal opinions about what you should do or not do about specific things out of the mix, but I guess that you would ultimately be the judge of that. I feel like although this book should have (hopefully) given you some real expectations during pregnancy, giving birth, and your first couple years of being a mother. This last chapter is going to be a little bit different than the rest of them, as it's coming from my own personal mouth. There is no research behind what I am about to say – just pure motherly advice coming straight from the heart at ya.

First things first – nothing, and I mean *nothing,* will go according to how you plan it once you have children. Ask almost any parent that you encounter, and I have no doubt that majority of them will agree with me on that. You can prepare as much as you want – whether it's a big travelling trip that you need to pack for, or if it's just a simple trip to the mall to do some shopping – nothing will prepare you for what could, or couldn't, happen before, during, or after what you have planned. For instance, having your kids all ready and looking spiffy to take some Christmas photos with Santa, and you are thinking that everything is going smoothly… until you arrive to the place, get your spiffy-looking, adorable bundle of joy out of the car seat, and realize that they have shit going all the up their back to their shoulders. Now, sure, you probably have a diaper bag with wipes and diapers, and you may even be prepared enough to have an extra pair of clothes in your diaper bag or car… but, did you bring an extra change of those spiffy clothes that your baby was supposed to wear in the Santa photos? My guess would be, probably not. It could be something as simple as taking your son to school one morning, getting to school, pulling into the parking lot, and him upchucking the previous day's lunch all over himself! *Nothing goes according to plan.* And that brings me to my next point: plan for the best, but expect the worst. I know – you are probably used to hearing "hope for the best, expect the worst," but in the case of motherhood, no hunny… it's all about that preparation. Do your best to prepare; and, if there ever comes a time when you are not prepared for whatever the hell just happened, the mom guilt tends to be a little bit less intrusive when you feel like you did all that you could to be as prepared as possible. But let's be real – even the best moms, on their best days, forget things. Mom Brain is totally real! Us mothers have so much going on in our brains at one time, that it is no surprise that things are forgotten sometimes. In our vehicle, I will leave one bag packed in the trunk that contains extra diapers, an extra pack of wipes, and a pair of extra clothes for each of my sons. Now it has gotten to the point where I need to stock up my vehicle like an Uber apparently, and have snacks and cold refreshments to offer the crotch gremlins! As with anything, you will go through trial and error and find what works or does not work for you and your family. My youngest son is prescribed special medication that has to be taken every twelve hours; so, in order to be as prepared as possible, I have his main prescription bottle at home, as well as a smaller one with an extra oral syringe in my diaper bag. I do this, because I have learned that I am not always going to be home during those twelve-hour timeframes in which I have to administer my son's medicine. Like I said, it's the small things. It is trying to think ahead to the best of your abilities. If you are planning to go somewhere with your children after work and do not plan on being home until later in the evening and probably after bedtime, try to plan to bring your kiddo's pajamas to change into, so that way you can easily transfer them from car seat to bed when you get home without any hassle of getting changed out of their clothes.

Speaking of bodily fluids and being prepared… as a parent in general, just *know* that you will eventually get every single type of bodily fluid on you. I had a baby that would constantly get spit-up all over me, to the point where I would have to do loads of laundry every other day between my clothes and his clothes having spit-up all over them. I have had a baby that started shitting in the bathtub and has yet to stop! I cannot tell you the number of times I have had to pick up puke out of car seats, off of floors, out of sheets… It's super fun *(…she said very sarcastically)*. Having a weak stomach will do you absolutely no good as a mother. And unfortunately, typically it is *always* Mama that ends up getting tasked with the job of clean-up. I would definitely learn how to not have a weak stomach… somehow! And, whether you like it or not, if you end up having a son, well… the pee will just *go*. Definitely have some type of plan to execute in the event that pee ends up squirting all over the place while changing a diaper. Fun little fact: they actually make these tee-pee things to put over your son's manhood while changing a diaper… but truth be told, I'm not sure how effective it would be! It isn't like you get some kind of warning that it's about to happen! Now, again, we come back to that word we just talked about… say it with me: *preparation.*

After becoming a mother, life obviously changes. *So much* changes. It is literally like this entirely new world that you were born into and were told to figure out how to navigate without any type of guide or map. I talked about romantic relationships in previous chapters, but I wanted to touch on a different kind of relationship that I would assume almost everyone has – platonic friendships. Now, whether your friend that you just met a few months ago that you are clicking with comes to your mind immediately when I mentioned those words, or your best friend that you would consider another appendage on your body comes to your mind… these platonic friendships change, too. And the words that I am about to say will apply to friendships, old and new. Your world shifts to focus on your babies when you become a mother; unfortunately, unless otherwise in your face on a regular basis, friendships tend to take the backseat and somehow lose the priority that they may have once held. It isn't that the friendship became less important, or you do not enjoy being friends with this person… it's just that being a mother takes up a lot of your time and energy. After spending all day catering to a newborn or perhaps a sick toddler, the last thing on our mind is usually everyone outside of the current four walls. Like I said, us mamas have so much going on in our minds at one time… and for a lot of people! Mamas are not responsible only for themselves, but now a child as well. And let's be real here – without us women, men would not know their ass from their head on any given day, so women typically take on the mental load of the man's important stuff, too. You will lose time for yourself, nonetheless anyone else that isn't your child. As a mama, it is important to remember that those that love you (and your child) will gladly ride the waves alongside you. Any relationship takes effort – romantic or platonic. Part of indulging in self-care would be recognizing that you need to have connection to the you that existed before the mama you was created. There are also the friends that may have been part of your life for some time, that you just view differently after becoming a mother. If you feel like a friend of yours is not a good influence on you and/or your family, you will ultimately choose what's best for the greater good of the family, and that friend will probably cease to have a place in your new life. On the contrary, you will also begin to meet a plethora of new friends… and yes, they are usually moms too! Going to play dates and finding mamas that have a baby around the same age as yours, has similar interests as you, and the kids get along is such a great experience to have! You will start learning more about yourself, as an individual and as a mother. The mama friendships that you create, I feel, helps mold you into the mother that you will end up becoming.

Navigating how to be a mom, a daughter, a friend, a spouse, a sibling, a niece, an employee, etc. seems like such a terrifying feat when you look at it from the outside looking in. And, in all honesty, it kind of is. But it isn't as bad as you may think. My biggest piece of advice to you in learning how to navigate it all – and doing so while trying to find yourself as a new mother – would be to give yourself some grace. Do not be so harsh on yourself if you feel like you are incapable of maintaining relationships in your life that are not in your immediate four walls, or if you want to stop working entirely after having a baby and never wanting to leave its side. Choose you, and choose your family. *Always.* You are replaceable in just about every single other area of life, except at home. Stand up for yourself; have a voice. If you feel uncomfortable in any kind of capacity, learn how to speak up for yourself and/or your family. And mostly, don't be scared if you feel lost and like you don't know who you are anymore. Know that it is normal; try to shift your perspective into thinking (and feeling) like becoming a mother was like you emerging a cocoon as a beautiful, strong butterfly. You will end up learning more about yourself as a mother, than you believe you would. Try to do it with grace… and boundaries.

"may the odds forever be in
your favor."

As all good things do, this too must come to an end. Our time together has been so fun, but it is time to wrap this up and prepare to get this baby out of you! I hope that none of this scared you at all when it comes to pregnancy, or giving birth… or being a mother. It is true what they say: being a parent is one of life's greatest blessings. Being able to watch your child see and learn things for the first time is like nothing that I can ever describe. I hope my book did exactly the opposite of scare you, actually; I hope that you close this book or shut off the technology device you are reading this on, and have a little bit more faith and confidence in yourself, in your decisions, and most importantly, in your body. I hope this book made you feel more prepared in what is to come around the corner, in any step of your journey *(up until toddlerhood, at least!)*. I also hope that this book will make you feel less alone. I hope that when you are up in the middle of the night with your crying newborn or sick toddler, that you remember this book and think of all the other women going through the *exact same thing* you are – and guess what, probably at the exact same time, too! Like I said – we are all in this together. Motherhood is like some really cool gang that you suddenly get initiated into when you give birth. It's all about finding your village… *and your superpowers.* And remember… never, ever forget to be authentically you – especially in the eyes of your babies!

Love and light, mamas.

References

1. *Human chorionic gonadotropin.* (2022). Cleveland Clinic. Retrieved January 16, 2024 from https://my.clevelandclinic.org/health/articles/22489-human-chorionic-gonadotropin
2. *Common tests during pregnancy.* (n.d.). John Hopkins Medicine. Retrieved January 16, 2024 from https://www.hopkinsmedicine.org/health/wellness-and-prevention/the-first-trimester
3. Wisely, R. (2020, Oct. 13). *5 Placenta Issues Every Woman Should Know.* Michigan Medicine. Retrieved January 16, 2024 from https://www.michiganmedicine.org/health-lab/5-placenta-issues-every-woman-should-know
4. *Chiropractic care during pregnancy.* (n.d.). American Pregnancy Association. Retrieved January 16, 2024 from https://americanpregnancy.org/healthy-pregnancy/pregnancy-health-wellness/chiropractic-care-during-pregnancy/
5. Marcin, A. (2022, Jan. 31). *What is the Webster Method?* Healthline. Retrieved January 16, 2024 from https://www.healthline.com/health/pregnancy/webster-technique#takeaway
6. *Midwife vs. OB-GYN: What's the difference and how do you choose for pregnancy care?* (n.d.). HealthPartners. Retrieved January 16, 2024 from https://www.healthpartners.com/blog/midwife-vs-obgyn-whats-the-difference/
7. *Group B Strep and Pregnancy.* (2023, May). The American College of Obstetricians and Gynecologists. Retrieved January 16, 2024 from https://www.acog.org/womens-health/faqs/group-b-strep-and-pregnancy
8. *Membrane sweep.* (n.d.). Cleveland Clinic. Retrieved January 16, 2024 from https://my.clevelandclinic.org/health/treatments/21900-membrane-sweep
9. *Medications for pain relief during labor and delivery.* (2022). The American College of Obstetricians and Gynecologists. Retrieved January 16, 2024 from https://www.acog.org/womens-health/faqs/medications-for-pain-relief-during-labor-and-delivery
10. Skowronski, G. A. (2015). Pain relief in childbirth: changing historical and feminist perspectives. *Anesthesia Intensive Care, 25-28.*
11. Lothian, J. A. (2006). Saying "No" to induction. *The Journal of Perinatal Education 15*(2), 43-45.
12. *The role of hormones in childbirth.* (n.d.). National Partnership for Women & Families. Retrieved January 10, 2024, from https://nationalpartnership.org/childbirthconnection/maternity-care/role-of-hormones/

13. *Is it postpartum depression, or just baby blues?* (2023). Medical News Today. Retrieved January 16, 2024 from https://www.medicalnewstoday.com/articles/baby-blues-vs-postpartum-depression

14. Salib, V. (2023, Feb. 14). *Differentiating Between Postpartum Depression and Baby Blues.* Life Sciences Intelligence. Retrieved on January 16, 2024 from https://lifesciencesintelligence.com/features/differentiating-between-postpartum-depression-and-baby-blues

15. *What are the most common types of baby carriers?* Chicco. Retrieved on January 18, 2024 from https://www.chiccousa.com/baby-talk/what-are-types-baby-carriers/

16. *The benefits of babywearing – and how to do it safely!* Happiest Baby. Retrieved on January 18, 2024 from https://www.happiestbaby.com/blogs/baby/how-to-use-a-baby-sling

17. *The Boppy Company recalls over 3 million Original Newborn Loungers, Boppy Preferred Newborn Loungers and Pottery Barn Kids Boppy Newborn Loungers after 8 infant deaths; suffocation risk.* (n.d.). United States Consumer Product Safety Commission. Retrieved on January 19, 2024 from https://www.cpsc.gov/Recalls/2021/The-Boppy-Company-Recalls-Over-3-Million-Original-Newborn-Loungers-Boppy-Preferred-Newborn-Loungers-and-Pottery-Barn-Kids-Boppy-Newborn-Loungers-After-8-Infant-Deaths-Suffocation-Risk

18. Scarff, J. R. (2019, May 1). Postpartum Depression in Men. *Innovations in Clinical Neuroscience, 16*(5-6), 11-14.

19. Pye, T., Scoffin, S., Quade, J., and Krieg, J. (2022). *Child Growth and Development Canadian Ed.*

20. Plant, R. (2022, Nov. 29). *Benefits and Challenges of Gentle Parenting.* Retrieved on February 10, 2024 from https://www.verywellfamily.com/what-is-gentle-parenting-5189566